The Great Stillness

THE WATER METHOD
OF TAOIST MEDITATION SERIES
VOLUME 2

The Great Stillness

THE WATER METHOD
OF TAOIST MEDITATION SERIES
VOLUME 2

Bruce Kumar Frantzis

Clarity Press
Fairfax, California

The Great Stillness
The Water Method of Taoist Meditation Series, Volume 2

Readers' Edition

For information contact:
B. K. Frantzis Energy Arts®
P. O. Box 99
Fairfax, CA 94978-0099, U.S.A.
Tel: (415) 454-5243
Fax: (415) 454-0907
Web Page: www.energyarts.com

Published by Clarity Press, Fairfax, CA

First Clarity Press Printing, 1999

Printed in Canada

Note to the Reader:
The meditative arts may carry risks. Individuals with medical,
mental or emotional difficulties should consult their healthcare
provider before doing these practices.

Out of the Sea of Struggle
Comes the Great Stillness

Taoist Proverb

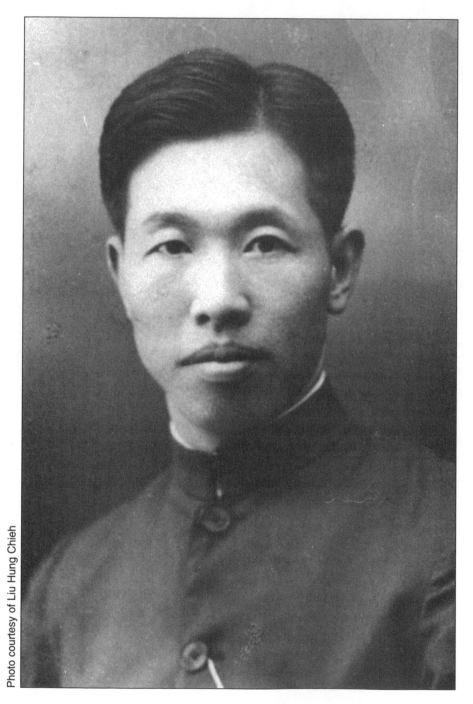

Liu Hung Chieh in his early twenties.

Acknowledgments

My profound thanks go to all my teachers in the Orient, to the lineage of Taoist masters which stretches back to antiquity, and most especially to the late Liu Hung Chieh. Liu's impact on me cannot be described in words, and without him it would have been impossible for me to learn and share the information presented here.

My gratitude goes to many. First to all my students, whose genuine interest was the motivation for writing this book, and who shared their invaluable insights on how to make this book particularly relevant to Westerners. To all those whose help and suggestions during this work's earlier incarnations made this become a better and more valuable book on Taoism. I especially want to thank those who contributed greatly, but for their own reasons did not wish to be acknowledged by name.

My thanks go to the book's editor Larry Hamberlin, without whom this book would never have been completed. I am also grateful to those who reviewed the manuscript at various stages and gave their input and help, including Frank Allen, David Barbero, Craig Barnes, Brian Cooper, Stephen Josephs, Kamala Joy, Bernard Langan, Dennis Lewis, Joan Pancoe, Eric Peters, Alan Peatfield, Diane Rapaport, and Bill Ryan. I wish to thank Jane Launchbury and Michael McKee for their wonderful artwork.

Special thanks go to the better writer in our family—my wife, Caroline, both for her invaluable editorial input and her extraordinary patience with me and with the disruption to our family life during the whole process of bringing this book into being.

Credits

Editor
Larry Hamberlin

Editorial Input
Caroline Frantzis
Eric Peters
Bill Ryan

Book and Cover Design and Production
Peter Schultz Printing Services

Artwork

Ocean Painting on Cover
Taoist Master Mo Dao Ren

Dragons
Jane Launchbury

Illustrations of Exercises
Michael McKee

Yin/Yang Wave
Michael McKee

Sitting Meditator
Michael McKee

Contents

Introduction

When I talk about Taoists throughout this book, I am referring specifically to various individuals that I have met in China and with whom I have conversed in Chinese. These people were completely immersed in the practical living Taoist tradition, practitioners of the various schools and subgroups. Many of these individuals were secretive by nature or were under political pressure and thus requested that their names not be divulged.

My reference, then, is to the living traditions of practicing Taoists and not to literary Taoism, which is often commented on by nonpractitioners and academics. The limited number of books available in America on Taoism tend to be filled with abstract descriptions or interpretations of Taoist rituals that never fit together into an integrated whole, or contain impossibly coded and baffling language, such as "the fire which burns the 24 embryonic knots and the 220 knots of the blood," or strange exercises whose rationale is never spelled out. In contrast, in this Water Method of Taoist Meditation Series, I have attempted to convey, in the clearest English I can manage, the practical foundation of the meditation practices I learned in China, especially from the Taoist sage Liu Hung Chieh.

The practical work of the Taoist water method proceeds in stages. It begins with preparatory exercises, which are designed to develop your awareness of the subtle energy in your body. Next come the middle practices, which have as their goal the attainment of inner stillness and awareness of Universal Consciousness. These earlier stages are explained in detail in this book's preceding volume, *Relaxing into Your Being*. That volume introduces several key concepts that are central to the present volume, making the earlier book a necessary preliminary for the present one. Moreover, it is absolutely essential that you have a firm grasp of the preparatory and intermediate work before attempting any of the advanced practices described herein.

Relaxing into Your Being concludes with a discussion of how the middle practices lead to the Great Stillness. The present volume picks up exactly at that point. Chapter 1 considers why, for Taoists, developing a full awareness of the energies inside the body is a vital key in the process of spiritual awakening. Chapters 2 and 3 focus on moving, sitting, and lying-down meditation exercises. Chapters 4 and 5 form the core of this book, an exploration of the inner dissolving process, the Taoist water method's primary meditation technique. Chapters 6 and 7 look into the area of meditating while having sex, employing and amplifying the energetic and dissolving skills of the previous chapters. Chapter 8 concerns internal alchemy, the advanced stage of Taoist spiritual practice. Here the spiritual infant must continuously transform the core essence of his or her being until, stage by stage, he or she becomes a fully grown spiritual being, capable of becoming fully enlightened, or one with the Tao.

The appendixes address specific problems that sometimes arise for practitioners. Appendixes A and B show how to avoid body pain or damage while sitting for prolonged periods of meditation. Appendix A covers how to sit in a chair to avoid back, neck, and shoulder pain. Appendix B covers how to avoid damage to the knees, hips, and lower back while sitting cross-legged on the floor. Appendix C answers several commonly asked questions by practitioners of Taoist meditation. Finally, Appendix D illustrates the main energy channels and centers of the human body which are relevant to the exercises in this book.

Before we turn, however, to the practical aspects of water method meditation, it is useful to explore why someone might choose to meditate.

The Taoist Emphasis on Health and Longevity

Many meditation traditions have for millennia served to awaken us spiritually and empower us to live from our natural birthright–Universal Consciousness. Though each tradition has its own approach, all of the more profound systems of meditation have certain central points in common. Because of their unique cultural and historical backgrounds, however, some place greater emphasis on certain qualities that in other traditions play small or nonexistent roles. Taoism, since its inception, has always focused equally on the pragmatic connections between the spiritual needs of the "soul" or "being," on the one hand, and the health and longevity needs of the physical body, on the other.

Taoists commonly look at spirituality and meditation in terms of spiritual health, rather than a super-ordinary condition called "enlightenment." Taoists believe that both spiritual and physical health benefit from ongoing maintenance and upgrading of the individual's Chi. Thousands of years ago, in his classic text the *Nei Jing*, the Taoist sage-king known as the Yellow Emperor (Huang Ti) laid the foundation of traditional Chinese medicine. The *Nei Jing* firmly establishes Taoism's living tradition of fusing the wisdom of meditation into traditional Chinese medicine and vice versa.

The Taoists also applied these same principles to aging well. The Chinese for millennia have used and been fascinated with Taoist chi (energy) practices, herbs, and acupuncture to enhance longevity and solve the problems associated with aging. Chinese tradition, both written and oral, is full of accounts of Taoists who have lived far beyond the normal human life span, the most notable being Peng Tsu, who in the imperial archives was reputed to have lived an extremely vigorous life for over eight hundred years. Taoists also remind us that living long does not necessarily mean living well, as can be easily seen by a visit to a nursing home and witnessing the barely mobile kept miserably alive by modern medical "miracles." More than merely surviving, the Taoists have always considered it important that the body remain vigorous, the mind clear, and the spirit at peace with itself until the end–however long that might be.

Partly because of this emphasis on physical health, Taoist meditation offers, on a pragmatic level, many benefits that can enhance other aspects of life. Among these are fitness and longevity, healing, athletic performance, decision making, and preparation for death and dying, as well as the classic goal of meditation in all the world's spiritual traditions–the realization of Universal Consciousness.

Meditation for Fitness and Longevity

Among its other benefits, Taoist meditation can help you manage the stress and anxiety that so often result from our accelerated modern lifestyles.

To achieve physical health and longevity, your meditation aim will be to awaken and balance all the energies of your body and to still your mind. An unmoving mind unencumbered by thoughts of past, present, and future is the ideal soil in which healing can take root. Without internal stillness, there can be no true rest or peace; in the absence of stillness, your mind will not hear what your body and spirit are saying. If you remain confused, excitable, and obsessive, your mind will tear your body down over time. The regular practice of Taoist meditation slowly settles your mind into itself. Stillness of mind can prevent you from engaging in rash or self-destructive behaviors that can lead to an early or nasty death.

Meditation for Healers

Because Chinese medicine has its origins in Taoism, many Taoist meditation masters have been physicians/healers. Their accumulated experiences and wisdom regarding the art of energetic healing pervade all the Taoist meditation practices. As such, the Taoist meditation teachings are thoroughly familiar with the various needs and energetic interactions between healer and patient. This accumulated knowledge includes an understanding of the deep emotions that accelerate, slow down, or prevent the healing process, as well as how healers can understand and prevent their own burnout by not absorbing the negative energies of their patients, or by neutralizing or transforming these energies.

The healer/physicians of Chinese medicine seek to balance the chi of their patients in order to heal them. The beginning, intermediate, and advanced practices of Taoist meditation empower practitioners to master their own chi and thereby heal themselves. The healer who through Taoist meditation follows the ancient dictum "physician, heal thyself" may ultimately (1) understand his or her own chi better, (2) recognize and comprehend from the inside out the nature of sickness caused by imbalance of energy, and (3) gain healing abilities beyond that normally possible solely by externally understanding and working on others.

If you are a healer, you will want to focus on those meditation techniques that develop both your compassion and your capacity to understand the basis of physical, mental, and emotional dysfunction. Knowledge of the inner dissolving practice taught herein will be essential. (Some other important areas of Taoist meditation for the healer are not covered in this book but should be investigated. These include five-element practices, aural control, handling the secondary energies of the body, and central energy channel practices.) The great danger to all successful energetic healers is an egocentric attitude on the order of, "Because I healed this person, godlike qualities must be invested in me." To avoid this pitfall, which can undermine your ability to heal others, you can use those meditation techniques that bring an awareness of the interconnectedness of everything, including your own self. The dissolving techniques, when applied to the results of your healing work, will help keep the focus on benefiting the patient, which is where it belongs.

Meditation for High Performance in Martial Arts and Sports

Just as Buddhists state there are 84,000 paths to Buddhahood, the Taoists say there are 36 million paths to the

Tao. Where many meditation traditions praise the courage of the metaphorical spiritual warrior, they abhor and are antagonistic toward real, combat-oriented martial art practices and lifestyles. One does not often see Christ or Buddha depicted carrying a sword or practicing physical combat. Among the world's ancient meditation traditions alive today, only the Taoists have embraced martial arts as a major branch of their meditation practices.

Many important figures in Taoism have been martial artists. For example, in Taoism the Eight Immortals hold a special place. Of these eight, two are martial artists and are always depicted wearing swords. Among these two is Lu Tsu, also known as Lu Tung Ping, whose followers are commonly considered to constitute the greatest number of fully realized Taoist meditators. Another Taoist immortal, Chang San Feng, is credited with creating one of China's most important martial arts–tai chi chuan. For seven hundred years, since the Mongol invasions of Ghengis Khan, the White Cloud Temple in Beijing has been China's most important Taoist temple. Its founder was also a renowned martial artist before and after fully immersing himself in Taoist meditation.

The martial arts component of Taoist meditation has little to do with today's television and cinema fantasy and image-oriented martial arts, but everything to do with the real ones where humans train and attain exceptional competence, delve into the core of themselves, and resurface with an unrelenting discipline and ability to endure physical, emotional, and mental tests and hardships. Taoists have observed that these qualities also mirror the deeper discipline and perseverance needed for more advanced spiritual practices, which can uncover the true essence of our being.*

Both in China and the West, many people are thought of as either "men of action" or "intellectual" personalities.

*B. K. Frantzis, *The Power of Internal Martial Arts* (Berkeley, Calif.: North Atlantic Books, 1998) explores this subject further in the discussion in Chapter 1 of the evolution from animal, to human, to spiritual martial arts.

Although Taoists have a fighting martial art tradition, they also have many other non-martial traditions that use chi gung movements purely for exercise and for developing chi, not fighting skills. In Chinese those forms of spiritual self-cultivation more naturally suited to "action" personalities are called *wu*, or martial, while those more conducive to "intellectual" or "literary" types are called *wen*. Although many practitioners fall completely in one camp or the other, some manage to combine both smoothly and powerfully, as was the case with my teacher, Liu Hung Chieh.

If you are a martial artist or a high-performance athlete, at the outset of your meditation practice you will most likely be interested in using meditation techniques to still the mind in order to counter any reflexive hesitation during actual fighting or competitive athletics. You can also meditate to open the psychic body's energy channels for producing greater physical power and for projecting psychic energy toward your opponent's mind. This latter ability can be used destructively to strike terror into another; it can also be used positively to project compassion and other positive thoughts. Stilling the mind is a necessary ingredient for you to bridge the gap, during competition and real or play fighting, between the physical and nonphysical (such as sensing the intent of opponents before they move), and for the most productive use of practice time.

When you learn martial art fighting or competitive sports techniques, the object should not be purely on winning or blood lust. Instead, fighting or athletics should be employed as a fast method to help you recognize and remove obstacles between your intent and your action. Through exploring the emotional, psychic, and spiritual roots of your obstacles and resolving them with meditation, you transcend the animal and human parts of your being. In the end, you learn to relax into higher states of consciousness and to function physically using higher energies.

Decision Making and Intuition

As life becomes progressively more complex, it is often hard to make decisions. Of course, if relevant information is available that can be analyzed, making decisions in a rational way is fairly straightforward. Often the waters of change are muddy, however, and a completely intellectual analysis of an unknowable future is not possible. At moments like this, using the inner dissolving process to remove the murkiness within yourself can open the doors to the center of your intuition, which otherwise would remain closed. Just as people throw the coins of the *I Ching* to divine the unknowable future, so the meditator reaches the same place without throwing the coins, by using the inner dissolving process and entering the heart of stillness within.

Death and Dying

For thousands of years Confucian China was a nation of ancestor worshipers. For the Chinese the felt presence of the dead exerted a powerful influence on the living. They believed the dead's anger and displeasure could come back to haunt those who remained and damage their lives. Conversely, they also believed the inner churnings of the descendants could diminish the peace of their beloved ancestors' afterlife.

In the water method of Taoist meditation, the majority of death and dying practices are based on the inner dissolving process. The many aspects of these practices focus equally on benefiting both those who are dying and those who remain and are connected to the deceased. Just before and at the time of death, Taoist adepts use the inner dissolving process to join together the fragmented parts of a person's inner being, so that they can reincarnate as a single unified integrated being, something that is normally possible only after a meditator has accomplished the Great Stillness.

At the end of life many people wish to let go of all sorts of emotions but cannot. They want to forgive themselves and others for perceived wrongs, reconcile themselves with relatives, friends, and enemies, be at peace with themselves and the world, and not take negativity into whatever they believe the next life brings. These individuals can use the inner dissolving practices to release and resolve their personal inner demons and ghosts, thereby enabling them to transit through the final phase of life in a balanced way and die peacefully. This allows the dying the possibility to take better care of their families toward the end and to release the need to engage in the reactive unconscious, negative, and vengeful acts that can cause massive long-term aftershocks of unhappiness after their passing.

The death and dying practices also enable the living to dissolve and resolve all the feelings and karma toward the dying or newly dead. This allows the living to finish the grieving process more rapidly, smoothly, and cleanly. Often people for all sorts of reasons do not grieve at the time of death, or do so insufficiently, and end up being bound by inner psychic chains to the dead, which can plague and disturb them for life. Years or even decades after the original death, the dissolving practices can enable meditators to free themselves from the unresolved issues that tie them to the dead and return at intervals to psychologically torture them.

Many areas throughout the world, including America, Europe, and Japan, have huge, aging baby boom populations. After 2020 these oldsters are going to create a dying wave of epic proportions. Until recently people died in bed with friends and relatives present; today most Americans have never personally seen someone die in their presence. The sheer volume of those dying in the future could again make seeing death a more normal situation, making the need for death and dying practices increasingly relevant.

Taoists for millennia have lived together in monasteries and various other kinds of communities. Owing to economic necessity and the need for mutual support, the baby boom demographics may result in large numbers of the elderly living together in communes or co-housing for mutual support. This augurs that huge numbers of elderly persons could regularly be seeing and experiencing their peers dying.

The Taoists have since ancient times viewed death not as something to be feared but as a natural event to be used for spiritual evolution. The energy that becomes available just before and at the time of death can be enormous. Group dissolving practices done during the final countdown and the passing can amplify the grieving process of each individual in the group–allowing them to release any bound energies both within themselves and the dying more quickly. The releasing energy of the contents of the dying person's consciousness helps release the parallel energies that are bound in the mourners, and vice versa. This helps everyone concerned to evolve spiritually toward an awareness of pure Consciousness. This releasing of the life force within–not with terror but with relaxation and inner peace–enables the mourners to more fully savor the wonder and beauty of the life they have yet to live.

Meditation for Realizing Universal Consciousness

Meditation was a main branch of ancient science for the Taoists and other mystics. The world's major religious figures, including Jesus, Buddha, Lao Tse, and Muhammad, as well as the yogis, medicine men, shamans, biblical prophets, and all manner of holy men, were also "mystic scientists" in the field of meditation. Their religious teachings are often simply verbal reflections of the living universal truths they themselves directly encountered during meditation. The living experiences came first, the words next. But belief and awe in the power of words became substituted for direct knowledge of the Universal Consciousness, the substratum that underlies all existence. If we truly wish to comprehend and follow the living teachings of these teachers/mystics from their perspective, then we must follow their example and meditate.

Meditation is a straightforward process, but it is not always an easy one. To pursue a genuinely spiritual life requires effort and diligence. If anyone tells you that achieving spirituality through meditation is quick, be skeptical. Meditation is not a free sample in some great spiritual marketing scheme. The more you practice Taoist meditation, the more you are able to relax and dissolve your blockages, whatever they might be. The more you are able to do these things, the closer you come to arriving at your own connection to the Universal Consciousness, whose intrinsic balance will naturally focus through you the qualities of love, equanimity, compassion, generosity, kindness, and wisdom. Meditation on your own personal consciousness (that is, the consciousness within yourself) and the Universal Consciousness, which are fundamentally one and the same, thus helps us to directly contact and live from our spiritual essence, rather than our selfish animal instincts and convoluted internal conditioning. Meditation on Universal Consciousness allows us to manifest our faith and our human potential, rather than just believing in them.

Although many traditions hold that the gift of becoming connected to Universal Consciousness can be granted by "God's grace," Taoists believe that it most commonly comes from the hard work of meditation, which creates the environment for grace to occur. Meditators will not be content to merely feel that they ought to follow the Golden Rule–do to others as you would have them do to you. Rather, each person delves deeply into his or her particular consciousness until it is discovered, beyond a shadow of a doubt, that one particular consciousness (that is, your own) and that of all others is the same. At this point you will be more fully able to follow the golden rule.

Meditation is not about religious beliefs, the supremacy of one religion over another, or about what a human should or should not do; rather, it is a tool to help you find–within yourself–the same spiritual sparks, the inner truths that the great religious leaders found, which generated all of humankind's religions. Thus, the meditation process is often experienced as a spiritual battleground. If you make a genuine attempt at moving toward the whole of creation through the realization of Universal Consciousness, then creation itself will eventually move toward you. That is the basic Taoist premise of meditation for realizing Universal Consciousness.

Meditation as Experiential Knowledge: The Cornerstone of Inner Learning

The world of science prides itself on objectivity and on knowledge that can be externally ascertained by methods such as observation or experiment. Within this paradigm, subjective experiential knowledge is looked down on as unscientific, anecdotal, and spurious. But genuine inner experiences simply cannot be replicated on demand through experiment. Consequently, most modern scientists invalidate the inner awareness of the human psyche that constitutes the core of the world's oldest major religions, including Christianity, Judaism, Islam, Hinduism, Buddhism, Taoism, and all forms of shamanism.

In the literature of all these religions one can find testimonials to central "mystical" experiences that can bring profound inner and outer changes. Taoist meditators, for example, helped to create acupuncture by delving into the inner world, locating the specific energy channels and points influencing health and well-being, and then objectifying their findings into a new science. Such discoveries are possible because, as mystical traditions in general suggest, all humans contain within themselves a microcosm of the whole universe. Mystical traditions often hold that if a human mind can penetrate its own consciousness sufficiently, nature will yield its secrets—in terms of both objective reality and the natural transactions between matter, energy, and spirit.

In the arena of "objective knowledge," we know what we know with a minimum of doubt because we can quantify and measure. But how do we "know" that something is real in our inner world and not just wishful thinking or self-delusion or hallucination? We genuinely know only if what is experienced causes a shift or change at some fundamental level of our being. Meditation is not the mere contemplating of an idea or belief. Often in meditation insights or creative capacities are unleashed spontaneously, springing from somewhere other than from logic or analytical thought. Moreover, many meditators are frequently able to comprehend complex body functions intuitively, through direct experiential contact with the most subtle interior levels of the body and brain.

Suppose someone does feel a dramatic inner shifting of some kind as a result of undergoing deep bodywork/massage, chanting, meditating, performing unusual movements, or some other experience. How is it possible to determine whether this feeling is insubstantial and fleeting or is actually a manifestation of genuine knowledge derived esoterically? If the experience has enabled a human being to access new capabilities, or if it forms a new baseline for appreciating or learning to live on either the secular or the spiritual plane, then chances are good that it is valid and life-changing.

Many times, such "peak experiences" quickly fade, especially if they are of a "Eureka, I got it!" nature. However, if they come forth as a consequence of prolonged, consistent meditation or other practice, they tend to gradually allow a human being to grasp certain phenomena in ways quite beyond the capacity of pure rational thinking. If Western culture keeps insisting that any significant "knowing" must come solely from the intellectual or the logical severed from an emotional, psychic, or spiritual context, then we will ultimately all be replaced by intelligent supercomputers. There is clearly something more in people than the intellect. It is the "something more" that we seek to know through meditation. Trusting what happens within yourself through meditation can eventually lead you to wisdom procured other than by conscious thought. It is this exploration, this inner knowing, that meditation has been all about for many thousands of years.

The water method of Taoist meditation and its inner dissolving practices have techniques for discovering wisdom, balance and peace of mind within ourselves. These tools are at the very least as relevant in modern life as they were in ancient China.

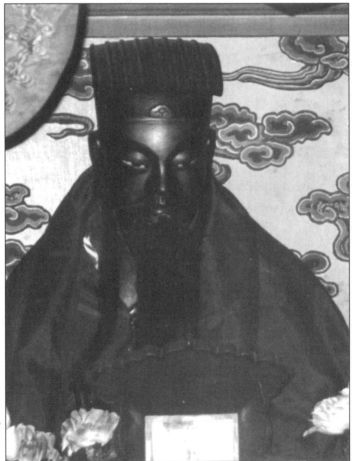

Photo by author

Taoist Immortal Lu Tsu, also known as Lu Tung Pin. This statue is from the White Cloud Temple in Beijing, China.

Making Your Body Conscious

CHAPTER

1

Lao Tse Tao Te Ching, Verse 39

Without the low
The high cannot be built

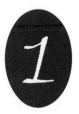

Making Your Body Conscious

Feeling versus Visualization

A central goal of this book is to teach you how to focus your full attention on the inside of your body until it wakes up and feels alive. This process is not the same as visualization. Reviewing an anatomy book and then visualizing what you have seen on those pages inside your own body may be helpful in the early stages of meditation, but such visualization has little to do with the practices taught here. The ability to feel what is actually inside your body, rather than creating a mental picture of what may or may not be present, constitutes a major difference between the fire and water methods of Taoism. Fire methods, which normally use creative visualizations, are more popular in the Neo-Taoist traditions, which were influenced by Tibetan Buddhism over a thousand years ago. The internal feeling methods, derived from the water tradition of Lao Tse, concentrate on allowing, following, and working with the energies that already exist in your body in each individual instant of time. Fire methods dwell on visualizing new energies inside your body/mind to create change; the water method, coming from the opposite direction, brings about change by allowing that which already exists in you to run its course to its natural conclusion.

THE WAY OF LIU
Reconnecting with Your Internal Environment

 Since I returned from China with Liu Hung Chieh's teachings, I have taught thousands of Westerners and am amazed by their inability to consciously and accurately feel the inside of their bodies. I have noticed that when people get a professional tissue massage, some talk about all this "stuff" they feel inside them, but after, they again regress to being oblivious to their own internal sensations.

We are all born with the natural ability to directly experience internal sensations, but in almost all of us it is lost before puberty. Why? Pick your theory: Is this a defense to avoid experiencing the mental and emotional horror of a previously experienced emotional trauma? Is it industrial society's inclination to reduce human beings to unfeeling machines? Is it a result of the emerging electronic world of image without substance, where sights and sounds are disembodied from human feeling? Or is it where "virtual reality" becomes the culture's new way of relating to the world with "virtual feeling, virtual sex, and virtual relationships"? Should we be in such a rush to jettison our humanity?

We possess "intelligence"–everyone believes that our brains make us "superior" to the animals. Yet if we lose our innate ability to feel the insides of our bodies as live, vibrant creations, we become inferior to animals. Taoist intellectuals recognized this problem thousands of years ago and devised solutions to enable individuals to regain the ability to feel the complete sensations generated from the internal working of the body. The Taoists believed that such knowledge was a most important form of intelligence and would allow its holders to deeply feel their personal relationships with others, with the external environment, and with the spiritual forces of the universe.

Why Does Taoism Focus So Much More on the Human Body than Many Other Spiritual Traditions?

Taoism is concerned with nature itself as manifested through the earth and the cosmos; it does not fundamentally focus on deities. This approach differs from spiritual traditions that emphasize being either blessed or punished (in this world or the next) by a supreme being or beings. Taoists see themselves as conscious individual cells interconnected to other conscious cells in the vast body of the universe. The Taoists say the physical body is real, it exists here and now, and for many reasons it is best to treat the body well.

If your soul belongs to your deity, it makes sense to focus on the nonphysical. You contact your God through your mind and prayer, a connection often viewed as continuing after your physical body dies, either through reincarnation or elsewhere in heavens or hells. In some religions, it is through sheer faith or supplication to given doctrines that you can buy the necessary postmortem insurance to create a wonderful rather than a tortured afterlife. What in many faiths makes you worthy in the eyes of your God is your innermost attitudes and yearnings, not the health and vitality of your body.

Taoist practitioners of the water school usually neither affirm nor deny the existence of an afterlife. They simply do not discuss this topic much because few (if any) have had reliable personal experience that conclusively resolves the issue one way or the other. Taoists are most clear, however, about the fact that we have a body and mind right now, and that Consciousness itself is knowable *in this life* through body or mind or both.* If there is something "beyond," it may be reached through knowing yourself at the core of your being.

---

* Throughout this book, mundane consciousness is spelled with a small *c*, Universal Consciousness with a capital *C*.

FOCUS ON A SPECIAL TOPIC
The Taoist View of Reincarnation

       In their philosophy, the Taoists prefer to focus on life here and now. Neither in the *I Ching*, the *Tao Te Ching* of Lao Tse, nor in Chuang Tsu's works is there a strong focus on reincarnation. The Taoist view is that the energy of life is at death mulched in the energy of the Tao and spun out again as another new living manifestation. Chuang Tsu, for example, says: "How marvelous the Creator (the Tao) is! What is he going to make of you next? Where is he going to send you? Will he make you into a rat's liver? Will he make you into a bug's arm?"*

Many Taoists believe that the vast majority of human beings do not have the capacity to reincarnate intact. They believe that when a soul dies, its consciousness breaks up and later combines with parts of other fragmented souls, thereby reincarnating as a mosaic soul. This idea is also represented in other traditions, especially shamanic ones, where it is held that a human's body can be composed from different past lives of various entities. Thus, some Taoists believe that the human desire to become integrated is based on a literal need.

The primary spiritual purpose of the preparatory and intermediate chi practices of Taoist meditation for achieving spiritual maturity involves gathering all the energies of an individual into one integrated, whole energy or consciousness. This unified energy/consciousness creates a *ling*, the Chinese word for "soul." A unified ling can reincarnate intact; a fragmented or nonintegrated human consciousness cannot.

Since many Taoists believe that most people will not come back as a unified being, they consider talking about reincarnation to be a waste of time. They do, though, discuss karma, which they often characterize as the Law of Return. In this concept, the energy you put out eventually comes back to you in some form, though it is not certain when or how that will happen. Responsibility for the deeds you do and the psychic energy you put out is critical to the Taoist philosophy of how life and justice works.

The life-affirming Taoists seek a primal route to experiencing the nature of the nontemporal "soul" by training the

*Chuang Tsu, *Basic Writings*, trans. Burton Watson (New York: Columbia University Press, 1964), p. 81.

FOCUS ON A SPECIAL TOPIC
The Taoist View of Reincarnation (continued)

body to be fully conscious and aware. By placing attention on the living human body and on Consciousness (which they deem to be immortal), Taoists hold that focusing on this present life is as equally important as giving credence to the concept of an afterlife.

Taoists Emphasize Internal Feeling of the Body

Taoists believe that sentient beings alone have the ability to feel themselves in a heavy gravitational field, such as the one we have here on earth. To take full advantage of this situation, Taoists initially emphasize body practices that are based on actual feeling rather than on such purely mental processes as visualization. There are many in all cultures who essentially ignore their bodies, who cannot actually feel the functioning of their bodies, and who live their lives totally in their heads.

In today's world, this problem is sadly becoming intensified as greater percentages of the population seek out cyberspace, where virtual reality is touted as looking better and more seductive than real life. In an emerging cyberspace culture, wherein people maintain that "virtual sex is better than real sex," a Taoist-like emphasis on making the body fully alive can be a beneficial counterbalance to humans becoming ever more physically numb and unaware.

Taoists have always placed great significance on physical sensation and on directly experiencing the Consciousness locked inside the body, which is absent in cyberspace. They believe that awareness at the cellular level is required to complete the process of fully integrating all eight energy bodies.* In fact, for Taoists, owning a physical body allows humans an unparalleled opportunity to integrate all of the eight energy bodies, a virtually impossible accomplishment for an entity in a noncorporeal state.

When individuals begin to get extremely sensitized to the inner balances of their own bodies, they naturally begin to become personally aware of, and interested in, the balance of their external environment–the body of Mother Earth. If this awareness can grow and be translated into action among people with economic power, there may be real hope for preserving our ecological environment, now seriously endangered by greed, rampant technology, and overpopulation.

The Difference between Using the Body to Liberate Consciousness and Wanting to Feel Good

From their ongoing observations of humankind, Taoists concluded that most people were not interested in directly understanding the Consciousness residing in the body, but only in feeling better. This conclusion presented a challenge: How could their tradition ultimately get people to become both spiritually clear and physically healthy? After all, the very heart of Taoist work, the point of it all, was to provide people a way to become aware of pure Consciousness itself; that is, Consciousness *without any content* (thought or other mental activity). For millennia, this effort was the foundation of their spiritual tradition. Certainly, in China there have always been sufficient numbers of intelligent and successful people who had seen what life had to offer and wanted to get at the root of things, who possessed a genuine interest in the nature of Consciousness and the Tao itself. However, the majority of Chinese interested in Taoism were those whose interest was

*For a description of the eight energy bodies, see Chapter 2 of *Relaxing into Your Being*, Vol. 1 of this Water Method of Taoist Meditation Series.

confined to functioning better in body, emotions, and mind. Taoists hoped that if they could provide the larger group with the practical benefits they desired, then at some point these people would undergo some inner experiences that would turn their attention to the main goal: meditation on Consciousness itself. This principle has been wisely espoused by many mystics as, "First give people what they want, in the hope that eventually they will want what they need" (that is, connection to Consciousness).

Making the Body Conscious Brings People into Meditation Through the Back Door

Many men and women fall into meditation by accident. In one way or another, most individuals begin practicing meditation in order to deal with the multifaceted stresses and traumas of life. They want to heal their bodies or ease their emotions by introducing an internal environment of comfort, and by soothing nerves strained in dealing with life. If you ask people why they begin meditation, you generally receive a common answer: "I want to feel better," which can mean they want to get beyond physical, emotional, or mental pain, discomfort, confusion, anguish, agitation, loss of control, and so on. The preliminary chi practices of Taoism, as described in *Relaxing into Your Being*, the first book in this meditation series, are specifically designed to address this desire.

You may begin practicing chi gung or tai chi purely for physical reasons and then find (perhaps to your chagrin) that you have awakened unresolved mental and emotionally uncomfortable "stuff." The genie is now out of the bottle. For unknown reasons the suppressed unconscious neurotic patterns you have managed to deny for years may emerge, demanding attention. By entering into the energy of your body and central nervous system, you have accessed your deepest emotional and mental substrata. After dissolving deeper and releasing your limitations, you progressively feel better at more satisfying levels within yourself, and can thus cope with external pressures more easily.

Much of what tears us up inside is our animal emotions. We often overreact emotionally and can mentally churn with inflated ideas of our own self-importance, lack of self-worth, or feelings of revenge or greed. Our glands release substances that make us angry and depressed. By energizing or enlivening your body, Taoist meditation practices can enable you to experientially understand and control the connections between your physical body, glands, and emotions. How? The practices achieve this by (1) exploring the workings of these body energy and glandular connections through the basic dissolving practices, whether done standing, moving, sitting, lying down, or sexually; and (2) teaching how to stop the body energy from feeding the glands, which ordinarily cause emotional grief when negatively energized. The process is fairly simple: either our body energy activates our glands, which secrete substances that cause us to feel anger, frustration, depression, and so on; or our body energy goes to the brain and fuels a mental churning, in which case obsessive ideas start to go round and round, gradually picking up steam and ruining our peace of mind. Grasping intellectually that the swirling thoughts are useless nonsense is not at all sufficient to stop them. The energy of the body itself must be relaxed before the mental churning can cease. Such relaxation must occur because body energy incessantly feeds the thoughts, running on a separate energetic track from our "intellectual" capacity.

To stop these life-sapping processes, the Taoists emphasized becoming fully conscious of the body and its energies through applying precise techniques. These techniques can control and transmute the negative side of the animal heritage embedded in our glands, without losing the positive vitality our glands and emotions give us. They reasoned that becoming an emotional zombie is as bad as, if not worse than, being an emotional maniac or intellectual neurotic.

The Wonderful Accident

During the meditative journey toward feeling better and stronger, a wonderful accident just might happen. Either through dissolving, chi gung, or other meditative practice, you could find yourself "accidentally" moving into direct personal experiences of emptiness and Consciousness itself. These Taoist body exercises were deliberately engineered by the Masters to eventually make an accidental encounter with spirit inside the body extremely likely. The direct encounter with Consciousness itself always has a profound spiritualizing effect on a human being, no matter where, when, how, or in whatever spiritual or secular context it happens. When people directly encounter the universal truth of the Tao (as opposed to reading about it or hearing about it second-hand), positive, life-transforming change occurs.

Consequently, meditating in service of the desire to feel good can produce a direct introduction to the universal nature of Consciousness (meditation through the back door, so to speak). In Taoism, for both secular and spiritually minded individuals, the body provides the context for an awareness of pure Consciousness to happen. In other traditions, the context may involve a deity such as God, Jesus, Buddha, and so forth, a mantra, prayer, childbirth, or a prolonged concentration exercise to create a matrix wherein a person can achieve a direct personal experience of Consciousness.

The mundane physical human body, even though it is temporary, can thus become your personal door to the infinitely profound.

Making the Body Conscious as the Gateway to Universal Consciousness

When you decide to take on the meditative work of realizing Consciousness, when you go deeply inside, you will encounter only yourself, no one else. If everything inside you is pristine, joyful, and wonderful, no problem. When you plunge into emptiness, however, the energies of the psyche are often involuntarily released. Your hidden unresolved confusions and pains can burst forth with powerful force. Certain things can then happen. For instance, the energies of a practitioner's body can destabilize, resulting in physical problems without identifiable physiological origin. Or a person can become an emotional wreck, experiencing deep mood swings caused by past psychic residue. Or a person can develop incredible arrogance or a superiority complex. Or the mind can be shaken to its core. Or the psyche can unleash demons. The force of these unpredictable blows can become overwhelming. Whether gentle or severe in nature, these are the manifestations of "the dark night of the soul." Meditators in all spiritual traditions must undergo such tests to pass through into the light. Often these challenges cause practitioners to quit the course and not persevere through their individual difficulties.

Based on millennia of practical experience, the Taoists maintain that weak or unbalanced body energies can trigger these occurrences. By stabilizing the body energies, much of the physical, emotional, and mental shocks to the system can be mitigated if not avoided altogether. Therefore, the preliminary chi practices of Taoism clear the body of blockages and physically prepare the channels to comfortably handle the amounts of psychic energy that meditation invariably unleashes. They are essential as preparation for serious meditation work.

Making the body comfortable, healthy, and at energetic ease with itself serves as a primary buffer to the potential psychic hardships of freeing the "soul." This condition also allows the meditator to progress smoothly, circumventing the cycle of one step forward, two back, caused by psychic destabilization. It also allows the meditator to have a strong, vibrant, disease-free body, which aids persevering. If, in the end, your meditation practice does not live up to your spiritual expectations, at least you should have gained vitality and some stress reduction—not a bad second prize.

The Role of the Central Nervous System

While we reside in a body, Consciousness itself needs a medium for us to be aware of it. That medium is the central nervous system (CNS). A clear CNS spiritualizes and relaxes us; a muddied one keeps us stressed out and brings out our lower natures. All the Taoist preliminary practices, including chi gung, tai chi, standing, sitting, and sexual meditation, are based on strengthening, clearing, and transforming your body's nerves–that is, your central nervous system. Chi moves along two primary pathways in the body: the fluids,* especially blood, and the nerves (CNS). The Taoists hold that only by first dissolving the obstructions in the fluids of the body, and then the CNS, can Consciousness eventually reach directly into, transform, and free the cells.

The CNS is the conduit between Consciousness itself and everything you normally experience. It serves in human beings as the necessary medium through which you experience or distinguish between your perceptions, feelings, sensations, and thought patterns. The CNS controls how the outside world enters your awareness, how you are able to experience what is going on inside you, and how your perceptions communicated through your body act on the external environment.

The CNS does not float in some mythical place; it is in your body. It is the key to both feelings of well-being and the attainment of spiritual fulfillment. Consequently, in its pursuit of spiritual evolution, Taoism emphasizes body practices involving the CNS.

Peak Experiences, Consciousness, and the Central Nervous System

Often in spiritual journeys, people have peak experiences of Universal Consciousness. Sometimes the awareness

---

*Blood, synovial fluid, cerebrospinal fluid, and lymph.

of Consciousness lasts for only a few seconds or minutes, sometimes for a few hours, days, or weeks. Sooner or later, however, it fades. Why is this a temporary phenomenon? After all the hard work you put in or just plain good luck you may have had, why doesn't it stay? The Taoist experience is that the light of Consciousness is constantly emanating without end. Its substance is what ultimately energizes every aspect of our being (body, energy, emotions, intellect, and psyche). Usually, the distortions in the CNS are so strong that they block out Consciousness and prevent us from fully experiencing it. Some distortions are stronger than others. When one of the stronger distortions temporarily subsides for any reason, the bright light of Consciousness shines forth, exposed to our awareness. When Consciousness does shine through, it obliterates or diminishes other things that are distorting the CNS.

Peak experiences come in various degrees of profundity. Neutralize a little distortion in the CNS and you get a "wow!" experience. Neutralize a big distortion and you get a super "wow!" experience. Neutralize a huge distortion and you get an irreversible life-altering change.

Although Consciousness itself is constantly emanating, unless your CNS is completely opened and cleared, the distortions of your "red dust" will again accumulate and block your ability to access the Universal Consciousness.* Each time Consciousness does break through to awareness, a cleansing of the CNS will occur to one degree or another, easing the way to experiencing emptiness.

When the CNS is cleared completely, it no longer obstructs Consciousness. Then you can become aware of Universal Consciousness twenty-four hours a day. Before this state is reached, the degree of clogging of the CNS determines for how much of your life, if any at all, you can be aware of Consciousness itself. Thus, the CNS is one gateway to spirit. Since it exists within the body, the Taoists emphasize

---

*For a description of "red dust," see the section "Liu Explains the Process of Meditation" in Chapter 5 of *Relaxing into Your Being*.

all work that makes the body healthy and vibrant to free the CNS from the encrustations (prison walls, if you will) that prevent us from becoming fully aware of Universal Consciousness.

The average person does the Taoist body practices to gain physical health and vibrancy, to overcome the stresses and diseases of life. Though the meditator also enjoys these benefits, he or she gains the tools that make a seemingly impossible task–freeing the soul–less daunting, more practical, and possible.

FOCUS ON PRACTICE
Taoist Internal Breathing

 Taoist internal breathing is a powerful way to develop your awareness of energies inside your body. The following breathing practice, which is taught as a series of twelve separate lessons in *Relaxing into Your Being,* is here presented in its entirety. Internal breathing may be practiced either standing (as described in *Relaxing into Your Being*) or sitting (as described in chapter 3 of this book). Remember always to breathe through your nose unless some medical condition requires you to breathe through your mouth.

During inhalation, you will do three things simultaneously:

1. In unison, expand the front, side, and back parts of your belly, and the back (but not the front) of your lungs.
2. With continuous unbroken awareness, follow your breath from your nose, down the center of your body, to your lower tantien.
3. From the edge of your etheric body (the external field around you sometimes called the aura) consciously draw breath in from the rear, through the ming men point on the spine, and simultaneously from the front, through the skin of your belly, into your lower tantien.

FOCUS ON PRACTICE
Taoist Internal Breathing (continued)

On the exhale, again do three things simultaneously:

1. Let your lungs and belly return to their original position with the same or slower speed than they expanded.
2. Follow your breath from your tantien up the center of your body to your throat and out your nose.
3. Follow your exhaling breath away from your tantien, simultaneously back through your body to the ming men and forward to the skin in front of your body and from both outside your physical boundary to the edges of your etheric body. At an advanced level of practice, follow the exhale to the point as far out in space as you originally drew energy from.

Gradually increase the duration of your breath; relax your body's nerves.

Begin with two breaths and rest for a moment. In time, when you can do two breaths with continuous unbroken awareness in a relaxed manner, then progress to three, then four, all the way up to thirty. Once you can do thirty, you can then practice breathing as a meditation and stress release exercise that will also improve your health. How much you want to practice after thirty breaths is a purely personal decision.

This practice is an excellent, simple method of learning to discipline your concentration, consciously become aware of your personal connection to inner and outer energies, and overcome the nervous jumping of a monkey mind.

Moving Meditation Practices

CHAPTER
2

I Ching Hexagram 27–Providing Nourishment

Pay attention to the source of your nourishment
And that which you seek to put in your mouth

Moving Meditation Practices

Meditation for spiritual evolution and healing is at the core of both the Taoist monastic and secular traditions. Taoist meditation may be practiced in any of five styles: sitting, standing, moving, lying down, and during sexual activity. Preparatory standing and moving exercises were described in *Relaxing into Your Being*, Volume 1 of this series. The present chapter builds on that volume by introducing somewhat more advanced moving practices, which in turn are a vital prerequisite for the inner dissolving process taught later in this book.

These rudiments, when learned and performed correctly, clear out the blockages of the physical, chi, and emotional bodies, blockages that can cause considerable energetic, emotional, and psychic problems. Without opening them up or clearing them out, people are prevented from becoming emotionally mature. And it is virtually impossible for emotionally unstable minds (those that cannot take responsibility for their day-to-day emotional lives) to move into higher states of spiritual consciousness. Usually, such minds commonly would not be able to handle the potentially destabilizing repercussions of moving up the spiritual ladder.

Spiritual practice is not an easy task even under the most ideal circumstances. Natural hardships, obstacles, and frustrations occur throughout the process. Emotionally immature minds will not be able to persevere and will engage in unavoidable distractions. This chapter shows how to begin mastering some of the fundamentals in order to prepare for advancement.

In practicing meditation, expect to examine your life right down to its core and, through long bouts of transforming introspection, to build up your spiritual and moral character. Expect to expose your own shortcomings and dysfunctions, overcoming what can be overcome and accepting what needs to be accepted. Taoism is not looking for people to be perfect, merely for them to relax into stillness and Consciousness itself.

Although the early stages of meditating may be easy, its later stages are not. In all traditions, there is an intense period of painful psychological purification, sudden unforeseen whirlwinds that can press you into realizing the full impact of parts of yourself that you have repressed, often for your whole life.

You will fully experience the darkness inside yourself, along with numerous frustrations, self-doubts, and fears. Yet this purification, different for each of us, is necessary to free the spirit. A good teacher can be invaluable during these trying times. Whether alone or with help, however, this dark valley must be passed through. The spiritual journey requires both the courage and rectitude of the strongest warrior and the loving, gentle forgiveness and humor of a mother toward a wayward child.

During this journey, it is easy to become totally self-absorbed and oblivious to how "your trip" is positively or negatively affecting others. It is good to remember that not everyone is on your spiritual journey, and that interfering with others because of your desire to dramatically "share" your newfound revelations may or may not be an invasion of their space. It is also important not to be distracted from your spiritual journey by people who, for their own reasons, don't like what you are doing.

You may find yourself moving between focusing on the self-interests and needs of your small "I" and a living sense of the universal contained in all things, sometimes strongly feeling your boundaries and sometimes losing them.

As you go deeply inside yourself and uncover ignored or blocked memories you will, time and time again, become aware of and remorseful over the hurtful and destructive things you have done. Little by little, you will need to dissolve and clear out the residue that can cause you to repeat these negative actions endlessly, thereby freeing yourself of your bad spiritual and moral habits. It is absolutely essential to learn to forgive yourself for all your past wrongdoing and foolishness. As you begin to forgive yourself, it becomes easier to forgive the past hurts of others, dissolving and releasing the anger and hatred you feel toward them. This way is necessary for inner peace.

The road to spiritual clarity is not usually a pure heroic upward ascent. Normally it is a spiritual roller coaster ride with many ups and downs, plateaus and limbos. It always happens that just when you are riding a spiritual high and patting yourself on the back, something upsetting will occur, your emotional bottom will fall out, and it's back to the drawing board. You once again have to dissolve and resolve your character's moral weak points or release long-buried traumas.

At times you will feel elated, at other times dejected and rudderless. Humans are not perfect, and it is not realistic to expect perfection in our practice. You will need to have patience and perseverance, and guard against complacency. As you release the darker sides of your character, your good points and then your inner joy and peace will emerge with smoothness and ease. You may expect this spiritual roller coaster ride to last until your mind becomes still and balanced.

The *I Ching's* Method of Moving Meditation: Circle Walking

We all need exercise. Walking, one of the most natural and beneficial forms of whole-body exercise, is loved by many. It is most enjoyable to walk out of doors in a quiet, beautiful setting when the weather is ideal. Weather is often inclement, however, and many urban landscapes are anything but calm. Though best done outside, the circle-walking meditation described here will satisfy the physical need for exercise even if done indoors in a small apartment. You can walk for a few minutes or over an hour if you so desire.

Even more ancient than tai chi, this circle-walking method was developed in Taoist monasteries over four thousand years ago and is the forerunner of today's internal martial art called *ba gua chang*.* Circle walking is practiced for three intertwined primary purposes. The first is to achieve stillness of mind. The second is to generate a strong, healthy, disease-free body, with relaxed nerves and great stamina, which Taoist monks needed both for normal daily work and to be able to meditate for prolonged periods. The third purpose is to develop balance and, perhaps more importantly, the ability to maintain balance internally while either your inner world or the events of the external world are changing, often faster than you can keep up with.

Throughout all the straight-line and circle-walking moving meditation techniques, do your best to implement the internal body alignments described in the standing meditation exercise taught in Chapter 5 of *Relaxing into Your Being*. Remember especially to keep your spine straight and your head up.

Methods of Stepping

There are two fundamental methods of stepping to be considered. The first is classically called "mud stepping" or "mud walking"; the second is heel-toe stepping.

The mud-stepping method is good for individuals with an intrinsic sense of natural balance and for those without leg or back injuries.

---

*For more information on ba gua chang, see B. K. Frantzis, *The Power of Internal Martial Arts* (Berkeley, Calif.: North Atlantic Books, 1998).

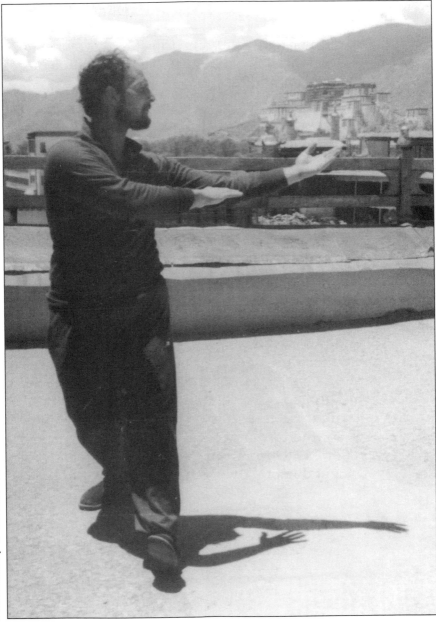

Photo courtesy of Caroline Frantzis

The author demonstrates heel-to-toe stepping in Lhasa,
Tibet. In the distance is the Potala, former home of the
Dalai Lama.

This is how to perform the mud-walking step:

- Stand relaxed with your arms at your sides, keep feet parallel, one foot one and a half to three inches off the ground **(Fig. 1a)**.

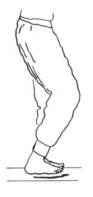

1a

- Step forward, keeping your raised foot parallel to the ground, heel and toe an equal distance from the ground. (The higher your foot is above the ground, the easier the step is; the nearer your foot is to the ground, the more body control is required.) During this step, your hips and body weight do not move forward **(Fig. 1b)**.

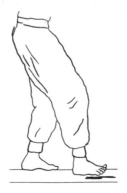

1b

- During the last 20 percent of the step, your lead foot simultaneously moves forward an inch or two and touches and brakes on the ground. Also during the last 20 percent, friction is initially applied on the ball of the foot with the toes, bringing the foot to a full stop flat on the ground. When you finish the step, there is no body weight whatsoever on your lead foot, above and beyond the weight of the foot itself **(Fig. 1c)**.

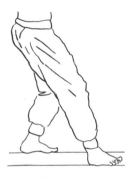

1c

The heel-toe method is more appropriate for those whose balance is poor or who have back or lower body problems. This method is essentially the one employed in normal everyday walking, only with more awareness than most of us use. Here is how this step should be performed:

- Stand relaxed with your arms at your sides, keeping one foot one and a half to three inches off the ground.
- Step forward with one foot and have the heel touch the ground first, making sure there is absolutely no weight on it.
- As you shift all of your weight forward, gradually roll your foot to the ground like a cat does, clearly feeling every sensation in the sole of your foot until your toes are on the floor.
- Finish with your weight on the lead foot.

Walking in a Straight Line

Choose whichever of the two previous methods of stepping that suits you, and incorporate your choice throughout all of the following walking exercises. Walk very slowly at first until you have a good understanding of all the various parts of the walking process. Then gradually increase your speed. (See **Fig. 1** on pp. 54–5.)

Part 1: Begin with your feet side by side and parallel, then step forward.

Begin standing with your feet together, your arms at your sides, and your right foot one and a half to three inches off the ground **(Figs. 1a and 1i)**. From feet parallel, your right foot steps forward no farther apart from your left foot than the width of your hips. Keep 100 percent of your weight on your left leg, and slowly step forward with your right leg, *without transferring any of your body weight forward*. As your right foot goes slowly forward and lands on the ground **(Figs. 1b–c)**, either heel first or toe first (depending on the method you are using): (1) maintain awareness of every part of the bottom of your right foot, including your toes; (2) be aware of every inch of air space your foot travels through, and every sensation, externally and internally, that the step generates; and (3) no matter which stepping method you are using, be especially attentive to how you put your foot on the ground. Try not to let the act of having your foot touch the ground disrupt your concentration or awareness. Don't get discouraged. Remember that your ability to concentrate will naturally grow with practice. In the beginning, it is a difficult task to maintain complete concentration.

Part 2: Shift your weight from your back leg to your front leg.

Keep your left foot flat and steady, anchored on the floor, your right foot ahead of it. Push back through your left heel to push your body forward until 100 percent of your weight is shifted to your right leg and foot **(Figs. 1c–d)**. Keep both feet flat on the floor. Feel every sensation as you push your weight forward–when you push from your left leg, when the shifting weight goes through your belly and hips, and when your right leg receives it. Feel every sensation on the bottom of both feet. The forward weight shift finishes on your right leg.

Part 3: Bring your back foot forward until it is parallel to your front foot.

With your weight 100 percent on your right leg, bring your left foot forward **(Figs. 1d–e)**, with the bottom of the foot parallel to the floor if you can (otherwise, heel higher than the toe, especially for heel-toe stepping), until both feet are touching side by side, or no more than six inches apart. When you finish, your weight is still on your right leg, and the left foot is one and a half to three inches off the ground.

Part 4: Begin again with your opposite leg.

You now will repeat parts 1, 2, and 3, reversing lefts for rights and vice versa.

(a)   Feet parallel, keeping 100 percent of your weight on your right leg, step forward now with your left leg **(Figs. 1e–g)**.

(b)   Shift 100 percent of your weight from your back right leg to your left front leg. You are now 100 percent on your left leg, zero percent on your right leg **(Figs. 1g–h)**.

(c)   Bring your right foot forward until it is parallel with your left foot **(Figs. 1h–i)**. Your weight is still 100 percent on your left leg.

Practice as much as you possibly can. Gradually, as your balance gets better, you can let your stride get longer. Your legs will stretch and your blood will pump more strongly as your blood circulation improves. Practice this straight-line walking for a minimum of one week to a month before attempting the next phase of circle walking. The straight line walking you have just learned will become the inside step of circle walking.

Figure 1 Straight Line Walking

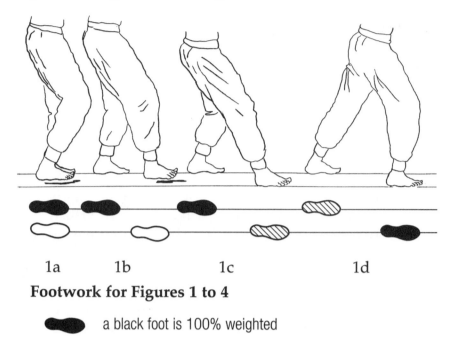

| 1a | 1b | 1c | 1d |

Footwork for Figures 1 to 4

a black foot is 100% weighted

a white foot is not touching the ground

a striped foot is touching the ground but has no weight on it

In figures 1a, b, e, f, and i, the sole, heel, and toes of your empty (weight-less) foot is off the ground, and parallel to the ground. Ideally the ankle of your empty foot does not flex, and your toes do not point towards the ground.

1a　Both feet are parallel to each other. Your left foot is full (100% weighted). Your right foot is empty (0% weighted).

1b　Your empty right foot moves forward without touching the ground. Your weight remains 100% on your left foot, ideally *without* your belly and hips moving foward in space.

1c　All your weight remains on your left foot. Your right foot steps foward an inch or two, as the friction of the ball of your right foot rubbing the ground brakes your step, stabilizing your balance.

Figure 1 Straight Line Walking (continued)

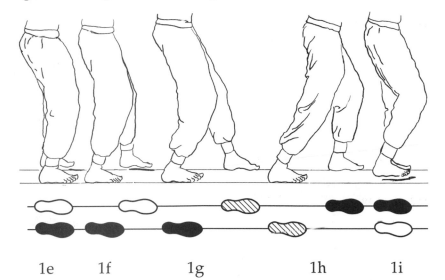

1d   You push your rear (left) heel backward into the ground, as your left leg straightens. This pushes your hips forward, until *all* your weight transfers foward to your opposite (right) leg.

1e   Keeping your weight 100% on your right leg, let your hips go foward a little. Simultaneously bring your rear weightless left foot forward off the ground until it is parallel to your full right foot. You finish in a replay of step 1 with lefts and rights reversed. From here to step 1i, reverse the order of the lefts and rights of the previous illustrations.

1f   Your empty left foot moves foward without touching the ground. Your weight remains 100% on your right foot, *without* your belly and your hips moving foward in space.

1g   All your weight remains on your right foot. Your left foot steps foward an inch or two, as the friction of the ball of your left foot rubbing the ground brakes your step, stabilizing your balance.

1h   You push your right (rear) foot backwards into the ground, as your right leg straightens. This pushes your hips foward, until *all* your weight transfers foward to the opposite (left) leg.

1i   Keeping your weight 100% on your left leg, let your hips go foward a little. Simultaneously bring your rear weightless right leg foward off the ground until it is parallel to your left leg. From here continuously repeat steps 1b–i.

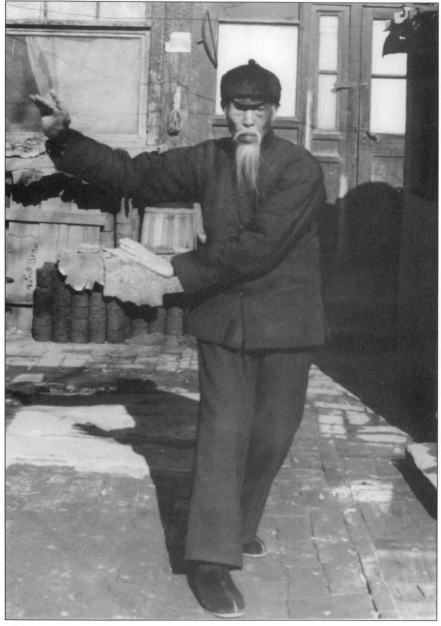

Photo by author

Liu Hung Chieh performs an advanced ba gua Circle
Walking technique.

Walking in a Circle

Walking in a circle brings up a vortex of energy from the earth through your body. Circle walking is a convenient way to walk long distances in a confined space.

Decide how big a circle you will walk and mark it off on the ground or visualize it within the space you choose. Beginners should walk a circle large enough to require twelve to sixteen steps to get around it. (Otherwise, there is too much twisting of the knees.) Fix the center of the circle in your mind or actually mark the center of the circle with an object, such as a rock. Now stand anywhere on the edge of the circle with the tip of your left shoulder pointing toward the center of the circle.

The Straight Step with the Inside Leg

Stand on the circumference of your circle, feet together, so that your left side is toward the center of the circle. Begin by stepping straight ahead with your inside (left) foot, keeping it parallel to your outside (right) foot **(Figs. 1e–g)**. Shift your weight 100 percent onto your left leg **(Figs. 1g–h)** and bring your right foot parallel to your left but not touching the ground **(Figs. 1h–i)**.

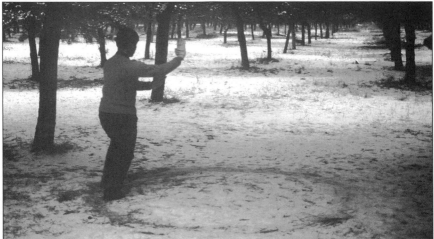

Photo courtesy of Caroline Frantzis

A lone practitioner Walking the Circle in a Beijing park wears a circular track in the winter snow.

Figure 2 Basic Circle Walking

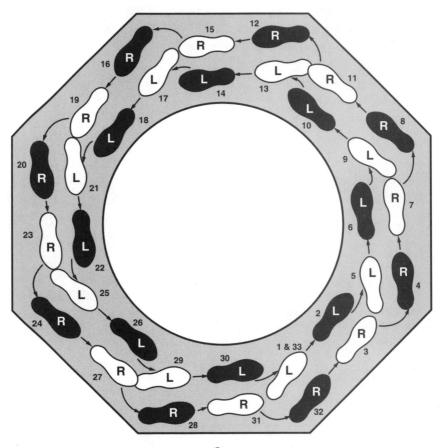

2a

2a   This octagon shows walking a beginner's 16-step counter-clockwise circle. The left foot is on the inside of the circle, the right foot is on the outside of the circle. A black footprint on the diagram represents a foot touching the ground. This includes the weight shift from the back to the forward foot. A white footprint represents a foot off the floor and moving forward. Step 1 is the beginning of the exercise. Step 33 is the first step of the second time around the circle.

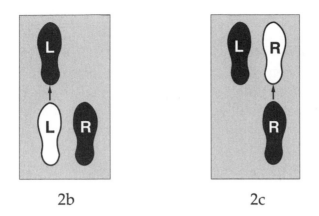

2b   2c

2b   Moving from feet parallel to a straight inside step—as previously shown in figures 1e–h.

2c   Moving from straight step to feet parallel.

2d   Moving from feet parallel to an outside step—outside foot curves inward, making an angle to the inside foot.

2e   Moving to feet parallel—curved arrow—shows the turning of the hips to bring the feet parallel.

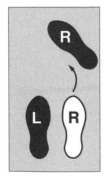   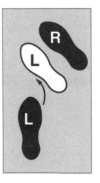

2d   2e

The Curved Step with the Outside Leg

1. In basic circle walking, the curving toe-in step is only done by the outside leg and foot. When walking a clockwise circle, after completing a straight step **(Figs. 1a–e)**, make a curved step forward with your outside leg **(Figs. 3a–c)**. Ideally, your inside foot should not move. As you do so, your outside hip and leg will curve slightly toward the inside, crossing the center line of your body and following the curvature of your circle **(Fig. 3c)**. The toes of your outside foot should move past the toes of your stationary inside foot. Again, you may use either the heel-toe or the mud-walking methods. When you finish the step, your weight will still be 100 percent on your inside foot. The curve of the step will be greater (60 to 90 degrees) and more difficult the smaller the circle you wish to walk, as in a small apartment or deck, and more gentle (30 to 60 degrees) and easier if you have more space to walk a large circle.

2. Next, keeping both feet flat on the floor and unmoving, push off from your rear (inside) leg and transfer all of the weight to your front leg **(Figs. 3c–d)**. (Your feet will not be parallel; the outside foot should be at an angle to the inside foot.) Be sure to maintain some distance between your inner thighs, which allows your perineum to remain open. Do not let your thighs collapse toward each other.

3. Now turn your hips a little, following the curvature of your circle. As you are completing your hip turn, bring your rear (inside) leg forward, until both your feet are parallel **(Fig. 3e)**, with toes facing in the same direction, weight 100 percent on your outside leg, and inside foot not touching the ground.

Figure 3 Left Outside Step

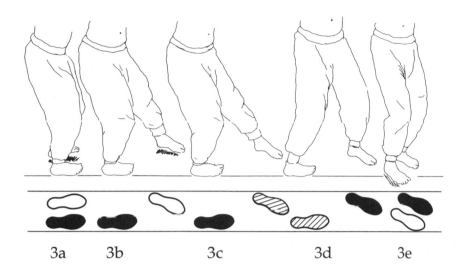

3a   3b   3c   3d   3e

4.   Repeat a straight inside step as shown in **Figures 1a–e** (See pp. 54–5).

5.   Your next weightless forward step will repeat step 1 and come out completely parallel to your back-weighted outside foot. Then continue through steps 2 and 3, and so on. In this manner walk the circle three times.

Figure 3.1 Right Outside Step

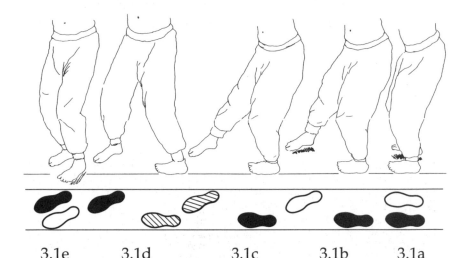

| 3.1e | 3.1d | 3.1c | 3.1b | 3.1a |

3a and 3.1a   When walking a circle, your outside foot is empty and parallel to the inside foot, which is 100% weighted.

3b and 3.1b   Your empty foot—which does not touch the ground—curves inward as it moves forward. Your weight remains 100% on your rear foot, ideally *without* your belly and your hips moving forward in space.

3c and 3.1c   Your weight remains 100% on your rear foot. Simultaneously your weightless foot continues its curving inward step, moving forward 1 to 2 inches, as the friction of the ball of your right foot rubbing the ground brakes your step, stabilizing your balance. Both feet are at angles to each other and *not parallel.*

3d and 3.1d   Both feet maintain the same angles as you had when you finished the previous step. Ideally neither foot moves about nor pivots. Push your rear foot backward into the ground to straighten your rear leg. This pushes your hips forward until all your weight transfers forward to the opposite leg.

3e and 3.1e   Use the turning of your hips to bring your inside foot parallel to your outside hip. Your next step will follow the procedures for straight line walking (see Fig.1) until your outside foot is again parallel to your inside foot and you repeat steps 3.1a–e.

Photo courtesy of Cosimo Mendis

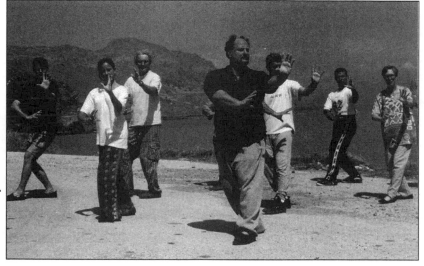

B. K. Frantzis and students at a ba gua retreat on the Greek island of Crete.

Changing the Direction of the Circle

Figure 4 Ba Gua: Changing from Walking a
Counter-Clockwise to a Clockwise Circle

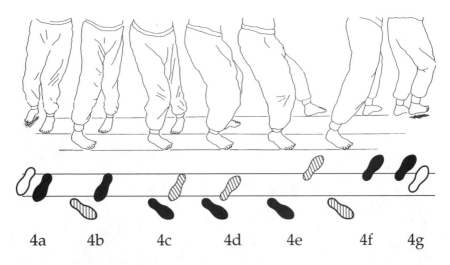

4a   4b   4c   4d   4e   4f   4g

Starting position: You normally begin walking a counter-clockwise circle—your left foot is on the inside of the circle and your right foot is on the outside of the circle. After you finish reversing directions you begin walking a clockwise circle, with your right foot on the inside of the circle, and your left foot on the outside of the circle. To avoid visual confusion, it must be understood that, even though the images of Figures 4 and 4.1 appear side by side in the diagrams, they are being executed at one point in the circle, as a 180 degree turn to change direction, not as a movement from one part of the circle to another.

4a   Bring your weightless right foot parallel to your left.

4b   Continuing your step, hook your empty right foot inward (see footnote on next page).

4c   Ideally shift all weight from your left to your right foot.

4d   Turn your waist and pivot on the ball of your left foot, until your left toes face behind where you started.

4e   Your left foot steps forward along the circle and brakes, becoming your new outside foot. Ideally, do not move your rear right foot or shift your hips forward in this turn and step.

4f   Shift all your weight forward to your left foot, ideally not moving your rear right foot.

4g   Slightly shift your hips forward as you bring your right foot parallel to your left. Your right foot is now on the inside of the circle, and you walk a clockwise circle as previously described. Figures 4.1a–4.1g on p. 67 will show the same procedure when walking the circle from the opposite direction.

After walking the circle three times with your left leg on the inside, it is time to turn around and walk the circle in the opposite direction, with your right as the inside leg. Here is how to execute the turn:

1.   Begin the turn when your feet are parallel to each other, weight on the inside (left) leg and right foot off the floor **(Fig. 4a)**. Then, keeping all your weight on your left leg, step forward with your right leg curving across your body, as before **(Fig. 4b)**. Now, however, let the whole leg turn in farther and cross as far over the center line of your body as is comfortable, so far that your right foot points toward the center of the circle. Your feet ideally should now form a 90-degree angle.* You

---

*It is not wise to make your turning radius so severe as to cause noticeable knee or back pain or strain in the pursuit of a "correct" or "ideal" movement. It is perfectly fine to turn less to protect your body's well-being according to the 70 percent principle described in Chapter 1 of *Relaxing into Your Being* (see also Question 7 in Appendix C). The least challenging turn–and the safest for your knees–is a 90-degree turn where your big toes are directly facing each other. This may progress until your moving heel can go past your stationary big toe. In the most challenging turn–and potentially the most dangerous to the knee joint for both novice and expert–your moving toes, after your moving heel has gone well past your stationary big toe, curve further and face toward your stationary heel at a 120-degree angle. An instructor or guide is required to bring you to this level.

may do this step either by touching the ground with your heel first and then rolling your toes down or by using the mud-stepping technique. At this point your right leg is on the ground and still weightless. You should feel no strain in your knees. If you do, turn your right leg less.

2.   Turning your hips, shift your weight forward until your body turns toward the center of the circle and your weight is now 100 percent on your right leg **(Fig. 4c)**. Turn your hips further around to face the direction you just came from, pivoting on the toe of the left foot **(Fig. 4d)**. Let your heel go backward to avoid strain on your knee and lower back. Pivot in any way that does not put pressure on either knee. (Note that only advanced practitioners do not move the left heel backward.) Your left toes should now be pointing in the direction you want to be going. At this point your body and left foot are facing in the opposite direction from that in which you started.

3.   Step straight ahead with your forward (left) leg **(Fig. 4e)** and shift your weight 100 percent onto that leg **(Fig. 4f)**. Then move your back (right) leg off the floor and bring it parallel to your left leg **(Fig. 4g)**, with your right foot off the floor. Your right foot is parallel to your left foot and one to three inches off the floor, or higher if your knees, back, or hips feel strain. Your feet have now completed the directional change: your right leg is now your inside leg, and your left leg is your outside leg.

4.   Continue to walk the circle another three times, now with the right leg straight-stepping and left leg curve-stepping.

Figure 4.1 Ba Gua: Changing from Walking a
Clockwise to a Counter-Clockwise Circle

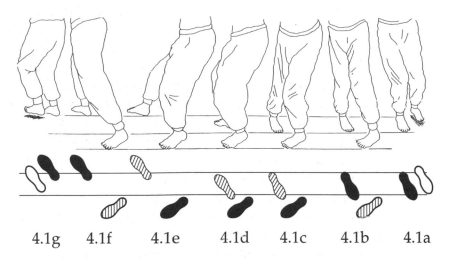

4.1g   4.1f   4.1e   4.1d   4.1c   4.1b   4.1a

To change direction again after three more circuits, simply repeat the previous instructions, substituting left for right, as shown in **Figs. 4.1a–g**.

From here onwards, pay attention to the simple but challenging act of feeling and being aware of your body during the entire circle-walking process:

- Remember that as you walk and change direction, at all times your torso should remain upright, without slouching or leaning in any direction. Remember the 70 percent rule.
- Keep your full awareness on your feet and how they are moving in space, millimeter by millimeter, inch by inch.
- When most people first begin, they tend to look at their feet, both for the sake of balance and to maintain awareness on the feet. As time passes, you will find you can look straight ahead and walk the circle with no need to look down.

When you can look straight ahead and be fully aware of your feet, begin to use your mind to dissolve your feet. You will initially find it easier to use the outer dissolving process described in *Relaxing into Your Being*.*

Finishing the Meditation

As you walk, pay strict attention to your feet and the space they move through. This will slowly bring your mind into a meditative state. As you walk the circle more, your mind will slow down and become quiet. If your mind begins to race, slow your physical walking down so you can focus on your mind becoming calmer, forgetting the day's events. Eventually, perhaps after months of practice, you will learn to forget yourself and enter the mindstream.** Then continue to walk and dissolve whatever arises in the mindstream. At the end of your circle walking, slowly come to a stop, let your hands come in front of your belly, and let your mind become as still and calm as it can. Let your energy concentrate in your belly until your belly feels like it is filling with energy. When the energy collecting in your belly becomes calm, you have completed this fundamental walking meditation.

*More advanced practices, which should be done under the guidance of an instructor, involve extending the dissolving process from the end of the etheric body below your feet, or even further, and then upward to your feet, legs, torso, arms, spine, head, and above the crown of your head to the end of your etheric body. A teacher is necessary to give appropriate and timely instructions and safeguards against the potential damages of consciously activating the body's upward-moving energy currents without adequate preparation. This situation is analogous to being fully prepared and knowing how to brake and safely turn your car at high speeds before driving in the direction of a brick wall at eighty miles per hour.

**See the section "What Is the Mindstream?" in Chapter 5 of *Relaxing into Your Being*.

FOCUS ON A SPECIAL TOPIC
Ba Gua Spontaneous Movement

 The ba gua circle walking described here is the beginning of a complete Taoist moving meditation method derived from the *I Ching*, or Book of Changes, the oldest and most fundamental Taoist text. In the *I Ching*, the primary or essential energies of the universe are represented by the ba gua or eight trigrams (*ba*: eight; *gua*: trigram.) This moving meditation tradition has existed side-by-side with the sitting Taoist meditation style for four thousand years. The circle-walking method of ba gua is said to have originally come from the Kunlun Mountains of northern Tibet. This primary moving meditation method involves walking in a circle.

Ba gua spread out of the mountains in the mid-1880s, when its internal energy development methods were incorporated into previously existing martial arts methods to create a new internal martial art, ba gua chang, which is considered one of China's most effective combat systems. A small percentage of the new ba gua martial art schools retained and practiced parts of its meditation system. The majority, which did not, consequently taught exceptionally effective fighting systems only, and not ways of becoming one with the Tao.

As a ba gua practitioner becomes more developed both internally and externally, he or she can experience instances of spontaneous movement. In ba gua language this phenomenon is called "when the dragon comes out of its cave." Spontaneous movement can happen while you are walking the circle. You may spontaneously start discharging energy in very powerful ways, doing movements no one ever taught you. You can have psychic experiences of all kinds. Until I met my teacher Liu Hung Chieh, I had never actually experienced spontaneous movement in the context of ba gua chang.* When I talked to high-level ba gua people in Beijing, I

*However, I had had such experiences in India as a practitioner of shaktipat kundalini yoga, under the guidance of Swami Shiv Om Tirth of Rishikesh. Kundalini shakti is depicted in the yogic and tantric traditions as a snake, symbolizing the innate force of Consciousness, which causes all chi and matter to manifest and can clear and release all the encrustation between your personal awareness and Consciousness itself. Shakti is depicted as the consort of Shiva, or Consciousness itself. In the same way, through the dragon, the will of the Tao is brought to the earth.

FOCUS ON A SPECIAL TOPIC
Ba Gua Spontaneous Movement (continued)

was told that only those who are involved in ba gua meditation have this sort of experience.

My first encounter with spontaneous movement was in 1981 with Liu at his home in Beijing. The period in which I experienced it lasted only a few weeks. One person who was watching described it as "shaking the dragon's tail" because my back and spine were wriggling so hard that it looked as if a tail was coming out of my spine. The source of these incredibly rapid yet flowing movements is the release of a human being's internal consciousness. In this process, your energy starts mixing with the energy in the surrounding environment and you can tap into the primal energies that give rise to each individual's physical existence.

A basic concept in ba gua is that you make your body into a "dragon body." The metaphor of the dragon, common in the West during the medieval era in Europe, is also appropriate for spontaneous ba gua movement. The dragon in Chinese thought has many meanings: it is the symbol of the emperor (as the phoenix is the symbol of the empress), of good fortune, and of higher aspirations and spirituality.

The spontaneous movements that I experienced were similar to what is called *kriya* or spontaneous actions in the shaktipat kundalini yoga tradition. The only difference was that the ba gua spontaneous movements took a form that is appropriate to ba gua and martial arts as opposed to an emotionally cathartic or psychic release.*

The chi manifested in spontaneous movement is called the dragon by Taoists in China and the snake by kundalini yoga practitioners in India. Ba gua dragon energy can be of three types.

---

*Years later in Taiwan, I again experienced a milder form of the dragon with students of the chi gung master Huang Hsi I who were doing spontaneous chi gung in central Taiwan. I saw all kinds of martial art forms created by people who had never previously been involved in martial arts. Both Liu and Huang communicated instruction in the dragon through purely energetic transmission without any verbal or psychological hints. Throughout mainland China there are now many groups that do spontaneous chi gung for pure health rather than spiritual reasons. If the cathartic component of spontaneous chi gung is overdone, it has been known on the mainland to lead to health problems from overstraining the central nervous system.

FOCUS ON A SPECIAL TOPIC
Ba Gua Spontaneous Movement (continued)

The first dragon is like the kundalini experience, where the earth's yang chi moves upward through the body and releases the consciousness. In the beginning, this often produces powerful, violently explosive releases of energy followed by clean, clear psychic states.

The second form the dragon takes is the descending of the downward yin energy, down from the heavens and into your body. This chi, which feels extremely light and amorphous, penetrates the body to the cells. You then experience the cells and atoms of the body moving apart (the feeling is as if cohesion between cells is being lost). You experience everything inside your bag of skin expanding, changing, and becoming amorphous without any sense of solidity, as your mind implodes inward.

With the third dragon, yin and yang combine as yang energy ascends from the earth and yin energy simultaneously descends from the sky. When they mix, a chi is created that becomes a living force inside your body, which physically moves you.

The spontaneous ba gua dragon movement is not a matter of having permission to move freely as occurs in dance, psychotherapy, and some chi gung practices, or combining previously learned movements in free form like a jazz musician improvising, but something deeper and more powerful that directly transmutes your consciousness. The Taoist dragon experience has parallels to, but has a very different feeling and flavor from, the movement of the Holy Spirit in Christianity, shamanic possession, or the spontaneous movement of kundalini energy. It also spontaneously produces martial art abilities and chi flows that would be virtually impossible to gain through ordinary ba gua martial art training, regardless of effort and strength of will.

The dragon energy literally grabs your body/mind and starts moving and teaching you what to do. This method of freeing bound spiritual energies is called "the celestial teachings of ba gua." These are teachings that come from heaven. It is not that you do a movement; instead, you are moved, sometimes forcibly. I clearly remember when it was occurring that I could spin on a dime in Liu's small room, avoiding objects. If I had previously done this under normal conditions, I would have knocked something over. Such motion

FOCUS ON A SPECIAL TOPIC
Ba Gua Spontaneous Movement (continued)

involved a level of physical coordination that even after twenty years of martial arts practice was beyond my capacities, yet I was doing it. My body was making jumps in the air that I could not have previously imagined. There was not any technique; it was just happening to me suddenly. After this period of spontaneous movement ended, it never fully recurred. I had to wonder if all of the kundalini work that I had done during the two years I spent in India, and that I had practiced for years, just happened to be coming out in my ba gua.

I asked Liu. He said that spontaneous movement had first happened to him when he was in the mountains of Sichuan and that it is a basic component of Taoist meditation. He was nevertheless surprised that it was happening to me so early in my development. When I revealed my previous kundalini *kriya* training, Liu said that my background had exposed me to these energies and therefore I was perhaps open to this experience at an early stage. Personally, my experience was that the Taoist method felt much lighter than the Indian shaktipat tradition.

Spontaneous movement is considered to be part of the spiritual side of ba gua. It releases bound emotions and gives one the ability to change energy to a degree that cannot be obtained from normally controlled ba gua practice. As these things start to happen, you can see into the root of what change in ba gua is really about. Spontaneous movement typically lasts for only a limited period of time, no more than a few years, and the levels of awareness it causes will not become permanent until the mind is sufficiently open, stable, and balanced.

Sitting and Lying-Down Meditation Practices

CHAPTER

3

I Ching Hexagram 52–Mountain
Changing line–nine above

Keep still with an open heart
Good fortune

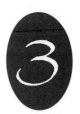

Sitting and Lying-Down Meditation Practices

The Sitting Practices

Sitting practices can be more powerful than standing or moving practices because, assuming your energy channels have opened and your body strength has grown sufficiently from the standing and moving practices, you can put 100 percent of your attention and effort into the nonphysical parts of your being. This 100 percent concentration allows you to tap into the mindstream much more directly, since you are disturbed by neither insufficiently opened energy channels and deep internal body imbalances nor the physical body sensations inherently involved in a standing or moving practice. Whereas there is a limit on physical stamina as regards standing and moving practices, sitting practices are virtually open-ended on this level. Some people have been known to sit and meditate for weeks on end without moving. The longer you can sit, the more layers you can strip off the contents that hide the nature of Consciousness from your normal awareness.

Sitting is usually a more direct and rapid path to exceptionally profound inner transformation than is standing or moving. However, after sitting has given you direct, easy access first to your mindstream and next to Consciousness itself, you can use this heightened awareness to enable the moving practices to be just as profound as sitting. You can also take all the standing and moving internal chi development techniques and apply them to control your internal body and energy channel movements while sitting motionless. This allows you to sit for much longer periods of time. These internal development techniques are taken from the sixteen-part Taoist nei gung system (described in Chapter 2 of *Relaxing into Your Being*), which is normally learned first in standing and moving practices for ease of assimilation.

Such a combination of sitting and moving practices will enable you to focus your mind on the tiny places inside your body where Consciousness is normally inaccessible and, by means of dissolving and then internal alchemy, transform and liberate your hidden Consciousness. The frequent side benefit of this is greater health and physical power than either sitting or moving practices alone can yield. The first and most critical phase of emotional work is done through sitting practices and the inner dissolving process, which is the focus of Chapters 4 and 5.

Body Alignments for All Taoist Sitting Practices

The basic posture for Taoist meditation requires sitting either in a chair with your feet on the ground, or cross-legged on the floor. Sitting in a chair is more practical for most Westerners, who generally have not grown up sitting or squatting on the floor as most Asians traditionally have. While sitting in a chair, keep your spine straight without leaning to the front, back, left, or right. To straighten your spine initially or when it begins to sag, you will find it to be more effective to lift upward from the front of the spine. The more you can relax the front of your throat, chest, and belly, the easier this lifting will be, and vice versa. If you tire and feel the need to bend your spine forward, focus your mind on relaxing the back part of your spine.

In sitting, apply the usual chi gung principles of posture, as follows:

Figures 5 and 5.1
Correct Alignments When Sitting In A Chair

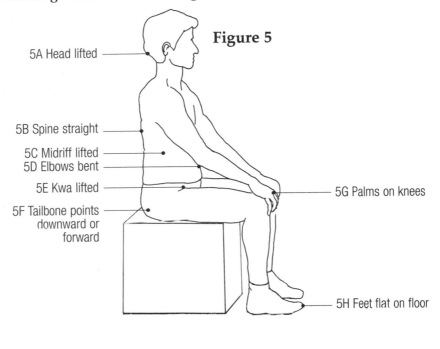

Figure 5

5A Head lifted

5B Spine straight

5C Midriff lifted
5D Elbows bent

5E Kwa lifted

5F Tailbone points downward or forward

5G Palms on knees

5H Feet flat on floor

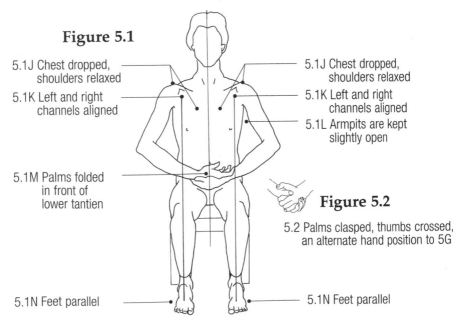

5.1I Central channel aligned
center of head is directly over center of hips

Figure 5.1

5.1J Chest dropped, shoulders relaxed

5.1K Left and right channels aligned

5.1M Palms folded in front of lower tantien

5.1J Chest dropped, shoulders relaxed

5.1K Left and right channels aligned

5.1L Armpits are kept slightly open

Figure 5.2

5.2 Palms clasped, thumbs crossed, an alternate hand position to 5G

5.1N Feet parallel

5.1N Feet parallel

- The tailbone points downward or forward **(Fig. 5F)**
- The midriff (the space between the top of the pelvis and the bottom of the ribs) and kwa are lifted **(Figs. 5E and 5C)**
- The spine is straight **(Fig. 5B)**
- The armpits are kept open, with the arms slightly away from the torso **(Figs. 5D and 5.1L)**
- The chest and shoulders are relaxed and sunk **(Fig. 5.1J)**
- The head should be lifted gently from the top of the neck **(Fig. 5A)**, and positioned directly over the pelvis **(Fig. 5.1I)***
- The body's left and right channels are aligned **(Fig. 5.1K)**
- The body's central channel is aligned **(Fig. 5.1I)**

The Taoist sitting position differs from the standard yoga or Buddhist sitting postures in that, using the Taoist method, you do not arch your back, throw your shoulders back, or breathe from your chest. Rather, the Taoist posture emphasizes achieving the natural relaxation of a baby. It calls for breathing from the belly, the back of the lungs, and the spine, as opposed to breathing from the chest.**

*This lifting is done so that the weight of the head does not cause any pressure or compression to the uppermost cervical vertebra. This slight head lift allows the back of the brain to remain unimpinged. If there are impingements, the messages to and from the brain will be partially blocked. Such blockage will often cause the sitting meditator to confuse neurological body noise with states of consciousness.

**Breathing from the belly and the back of the lungs is part of the Taoist internal breathing practice described in Chapter 1. Spinal breathing is an advanced form of nei gung breath work that is not covered in this book.

Figures 6 and 6.1
Incorrect Alignments When Sitting In A Chair

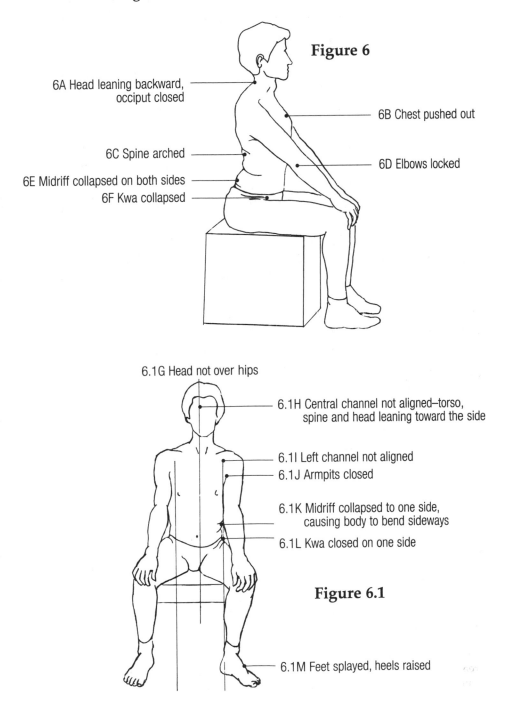

Figure 6

6A Head leaning backward, occiput closed

6B Chest pushed out

6C Spine arched

6D Elbows locked

6E Midriff collapsed on both sides

6F Kwa collapsed

6.1G Head not over hips

6.1H Central channel not aligned–torso, spine and head leaning toward the side

6.1I Left channel not aligned

6.1J Armpits closed

6.1K Midriff collapsed to one side, causing body to bend sideways

6.1L Kwa closed on one side

Figure 6.1

6.1M Feet splayed, heels raised

Three Basic Chair-Sitting Postures

As noted, to meditate the Taoist way, you do not have to sit on the floor in a full or half lotus position.* In the West, many people suffer from back problems or an injured or stiff hip, knee, or ankle, any of which can prevent them from attaining the full or half lotus. These conditions are so prevalent in the West that ergonomic chairs are designed for desk-bound workers to accommodate or avoid such physical problems. The critical goal for anyone practicing meditation is the freeing of the spirit, not sitting on the floor with your legs twisted beyond your capacity. The chair-sitting meditation posture described herein has been used by Taoist meditators and in times past by many Chinese emperors, members of the Imperial Court, and senior Chinese officials and magistrates.

Three Ways to Sit and Meditate in a Chair

There are three ways you can meditate while sitting in a chair.** These same chair-sitting techniques can be adapted to any type of office work, especially to work involving computers.

1.   When sitting in a chair, keep both feet flat on the floor, with the outsides of your feet being no wider than your shoulders **(Figs. 5H and 5.1N)**. If you can, rest the palms of your hands on your

---

*A full lotus position is one in which your rear end sits firmly on the floor, both legs are crossed, both knees are touching the floor, your left foot rests on your right thigh, and your right foot rests on your left thigh. In a half lotus, only one leg is on the opposite thigh, with its knee resting on the opposite foot or on the floor.

The chair you use for meditation should be one with a flat, unmoving bottom (not a canvas chair) with at least an inch of free space on each side of your hips and a solid, unmoving, straight backrest set perpendicular to the chair bottom. The chair should be the height of your knees, so you can sit with your feet flat on the floor with your knees bent at an angle of approximately 90 degrees **(Figs. 5 and 5.1).

THE WAY OF LIU
Thoughts on Sitting Positions for Meditation

Before my back was severely damaged in a car accident, I had no trouble sitting in the half or full lotus position for hours on end. Over a twenty-year span I had practiced stretching my body doing martial arts, Taoist yoga, and hatha yoga. For two years in India, like the Indian population in general, I sat on the floor, not in a chair, and I squatted to go to the toilet. But after my car accident, I found that owing to the shifting realities of body pain I could progress further in meditation by sitting in a chair rather than on the floor. Liu Hung Chieh, who was trained in the classic Chinese tradition, also practiced sitting in a chair as well as sitting on the floor. *You do not have to sit like a yogi to be able to meditate.*

kneecaps **(Fig. 5G)**, your fingertips ideally pointing straight ahead. Your elbows should be bent and loose, not stiff-armed **(Fig. 5D)**; keep your elbow tips gently moving downward toward your thighs. If you raise your elbows your shoulders will raise, and your spine will then tire more rapidly. Move your elbows gently to the sides. This move will create space inside your body where your spine can move easily and be more easily held straight. In an alternative method, place your palms along the body's center line, directly in front of your lower tantien. Your palms may be touching surface to surface with hands lightly clasped **(Fig. 5.2)**, or the back of one hand may rest on the palm of the other **(Fig. 5.1M)**, palms facing up (which hand is on top may be alternated over time). If at all possible, *do not touch the backrest of the chair with your spine.* Your body should be at ease, and your spine in particular should remain relaxed and straight **(Fig. 5B)**.

Figure 7 The Buttocks Support The Lower Back

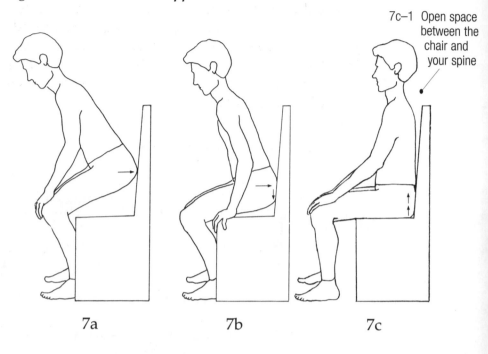

7c–1 Open space
between the
chair and
your spine

7a   7b   7c

2.   You may find that all of these unsupported back
            positions are too straining or painful for your back
            or neck. If so, sit back in the chair as you slide
            down the backrest **(Fig. 7a)**, and press your upper
            buttock muscles backward and upward to lift
            against the back of the chair **(Figs. 7b–c)**. This
            motion allows your buttock and back muscles to
            connect without gaps. The motion pushes your
            buttock muscles up against the back of the chair
            (Fig. 7c), thereby providing a stabilizing support
            for your lower back. In contrast, if your buttock
            muscles push downward into the seat of the chair,
            the muscles of your lower back can also be pulled
            down. A downward muscle movement increases
            the arch of your lower back, compressing your
            vertebrae and straining your lower back muscles.
            This progression can then pull the vertebrae of

your lower back out of alignment. So keep your spine straight, without any rounding or slumping. Keep your spine away from making contact with the middle and upper part of your chair's backrest **(Fig. 7c–1)**. Only your rear end touches the back of the chair to push your lower back muscles upwards, adding back support.

Figure 8 The Spine Flat Against The Backrest

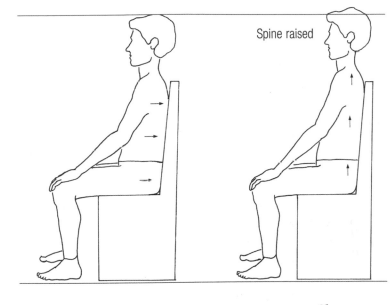

8a   8b

3.   If you still experience too much physical pain, then allow your back to be fully supported by the back of the chair. This is best done in two stages. First, as you sit consciously use the pressure of the chair against your back **(Fig. 8a)** to keep as much space as possible between each of your vertebrae along the whole length of your spine. You can use the adhesive quality and friction of the fasciae of your back to stick to the chair's backrest, similar to the

way a wet T-shirt sticks to your skin. Second, when being fully supported by a backrest pay attention, at regular intervals, to equally lifting and lengthening all parts of the spine **(Fig. 8b)**, with the idea of keeping the spinal cord lightly stretched and not compressed. Uneven compression of the spinal cord will eventually result in the back collapsing somewhere, straining muscles or causing vertebrae to misalign. Sitting correctly relieves these problems. Your sitting time should be spent working on your internal meditation techniques, rather than squirming or being distracted by physical discomfort. For more information regarding how to reduce or eliminate the pains caused by prolonged sitting in a chair, refer to Appendix A.

Taoist Sitting Meditation: Using the Breath, Vibration, and Ultimately the Mind to Awaken Internal Sensations

In the Taoist water method, as in many other schools of meditation, including Buddhism's Vipassana and Zen traditions and many schools of Chinese chi gung, the first and most commonly used sitting practice is to increase your awareness by following your breath as it enters your body. As you pay close attention to your inhaled breath, you will find that doing so over time will enable you to feel the chi that is moving inside your body. After a period of practice, through contact with the chi, you will feel the quality and movement of your insides, including blood vessels, muscles, joints, glands, internal organs, spinal cord, and brain. For example, if you were to close your eyes (to enhance your concentration) and breathe in through your nose or mouth while at the same time trying to feel energy breathing into your hand from outside your body, then sooner or later you would find that you could feel tiny sensations in your hand that you previously could not. By practicing more, the level and refinement of the sensations become such that you can eventually feel the blood moving through the vessels of your hand. Over time, you then can develop the ability to focus your breath and awareness and control the flow of blood in your hand.

Eventually, after much practice, you will be able to do without the support of your breath and can just use your mind to direct the flow of blood in your hand. This activity will eventually lead to a mind/body fusion, in which by relying purely on your *intent* you can directly feel and control chi movement within the body—the foundation on which all Taoist chi practices are based.

A second preliminary method used with variations in both the Taoist and some Indian and Tibetan yogic traditions involves emitting a range of both high- and low-pitched sounds to focus vibrations inside the body.* Vibrations increase awareness, and the awareness gradually leads to the ability to feel. In the beginning, these sounds need to be done quite loudly, so you can feel the vibrations shaking up your insides beyond a shadow of a doubt. By degrees, the internal vibrations become stronger while the sounds themselves become progressively quieter and ultimately inaudible, causing you to more clearly feel and differentiate ever more subtle sensations. These vibrations agitate the chi inside the body, making it easier to feel your insides. Breath work may be coordinated with the vibrations, or your awareness may focus purely on feeling what the vibrations touch and penetrate. Again, after these vibrations stabilize your ability to feel your insides, thus making your often hidden inner landscape more fully alive and consciously aware, you can next begin to use *only* your mind/awareness for this purpose.

There are a number of situations in which we can naturally feel the connection between the inside of our body

---

*As explained in Chapter 8, the exact sounds used by Chinese Taoists cannot be rendered phonetically in a way that an English-speaking reader can use. They must be learned directly from a teacher. These sounds are not the equivalent of mantras. They can be done simply as generalized sounds; in fact, you can make up your own. The point is to create internal vibrations.

and our external environment: for example, from our nose all the way to our lungs when we breath, from our mouth down our throat and into our stomach when we eat, from our anus during elimination, and from our genitals during urination and sex.* In the beginning, you can focus either on your breath or on vibrations, or you can alternate between them, depending on which makes it is easier for you to feel inside. After you have gained an initial access to the sensations of your interior world by breathing or vibrating your insides, you can then practice by leaving these preliminary training aids behind and concentrating on using only your mind's awareness and intention to penetrate inside yourself. Normally, some people find it takes time (weeks, months, or even years of sustained practice) to penetrate even one inch inside the body. Over time, however, you want to be able to progressively feel every cubic inch of space inside your body.

After practicing this mind-only technique, many delude themselves, certain that they can feel their insides when in fact they cannot. It may help to remember that once you can feel the inside of your body clearly, with some effort you should be able to move any given part of your internal body at will, no matter how slightly. You could simply have someone with sensitive hands give you a reality check as to whether or not your perceptions of your abilities correspond to what is actually happening.

In sitting meditation we start from such places in the body where we can feel something, then learn to feel further into the body, ultimately into all the places where we are ordinarily numb. Presented here are four techniques that can be applied to begin the work of going from the outside of the body inward.**

*Nine orifices are used in this Taoist practice: the eyes, ears, and nostrils (two of each), and the mouth, anus, and urethra. One other opening is at the crown of the head, at the fontanel, which breathes (opens and closes) in infants, but not in most adults without a period of training.

**There are separate techniques for each of the nine orifices of the body and the fontanel. Only four are described here for the sake of brevity. Depending on how open an individual's body is, varying results can be achieved in hours, days, months, or even years. It is best to learn directly from a teacher.

1.   Focus attention on your breath or any vibrations you deliberately generate into your nose when you inhale, and feel your physical breath move slowly inside your body. Follow your inhaled breath as far as you can on the inhale, then retrace your path back to your nose on the exhale. Practice this technique for a while until you can do it easily and comfortably with no gaps in your awareness, down your jaw to the base of your throat.

Continuing slowly but surely, over time, with concentrated attention in association with breath, feel whatever subtle sensations naturally arise down into your jaw, neck, arms, fingertips, torso, hips, legs, feet, and below your feet, where you personally connect to the energy of the earth through your etheric body. Do this in clear progressive stages, becoming comfortable at each stage before proceeding on. Next, follow the energies and sensations generated by your breath (pressure, warmth, cold, tingling, etc.) up from the bottom of your feet to the top of your head. Afterwards follow the breath upward from your nostrils into your head until you can feel the inside of the skull and brain and feel above your head to the boundary of your etheric body, where you personally connect to the energies of the cosmos.

Next, stop using breath. Progress to relying on only your attention and awareness to feel inside your body, following the same up-and-down procedures. (Some who are psychically sensitive will often find it easier to feel the energy outside their body, rather than the energy inside; others may feel the reverse.)

2.   Do the exact same procedures you did with your nose, only now begin the process from the mouth.

3.   Next, start the process from your anus. First move your attention down to your genitals, pelvic floor, perineum, legs, feet, to below the floor. Now retrace your steps up from below the floor to your anus. Next, you will want to go from your anus in a generalized way inside your pelvis and torso to the level of your heart and then, simultaneously,

move in two branches. The first branch is upward to the neck, brain/skull, crown of the head, and the point above your head where your etheric body ends. The second branch is up your upper back to your shoulders, elbows, wrist, palm, and fingers.* Next, simultaneously, retrace your steps back from above your head and fingertips to your anus.

4.   Beginning from your genitals, go down to below the floor and back up to your genitals following the same pathway as you did in step 3. Next, go from the genitals to the tailbone, up the spine to the occipital bone, through the brain to the crown of the head, to the energy point above your head at the end of your etheric body. Next, retrace the same pathway from above your head, down the spine to the genitals. Now upward from the genitals, through the whole of the inside of your pelvis and torso and spine to the whole of the inside of your body to the level of your heart. From there, move simultaneously to your shoulders and up the spine to the base of the neck and onward to your fingertips, the top of your head, and above your head to the end of your etheric body.

Then, at a point beginning at the top of your head (or above your head, if you can feel the energy of your aura), slowly feel your way down through your body until you reach your lower tantien, and from there go down your legs to below your feet.

It is important to *actually feel* your body and not to merely visualize its different parts. This process of internally sensing the body starting at the head and moving down to the lower tantien can take a long time; indeed, you can spend a one-hour session of meditation working on only a small segment of your body. After gaining experience, your ability to feel inside and penetrate your body with awareness will

*See Appendix D.

intensify. At this point you should be gaining the ability to actually feel your internal sensations. As you move your attention through your body, you will probably encounter areas that feel full of all sorts of internal content–things stuck, blocked, uncomfortable, agitated, happy, depressed, and so on. These and all other Taoist meditation practices ultimately involve dissolving and releasing the energy of these blockages, as described in the next chapter, until you become internally free.

The Lying-Down Practices

The lying-down practices are the most difficult of the five styles of meditation. To have your mind, chi, and spirit stay fully conscious and to practice for hours on end while your body is totally relaxed is not easy. In fact, you may become so relaxed that you and others become aware of your body's snoring. However, you are not dreaming, but remain wide awake. Ordinarily, the lying-down practices are not recommended until after a person has had substantial experience with the standing, moving, and sitting styles. Consequently, the lying-down style is considered an advanced practice.

The ideal state when practicing lying-down meditation is to have your body be completely motionless. Since you may be lying completely still for more than one hour, it is best to lie on a surface that you find extremely comfortable, one that is neither too soft nor too hard. An overly hard or soft sleeping surface will most likely prevent your body from relaxing completely. Overly soft surfaces will cause your body to sag, putting pressure from internal body weight on your bones, muscles, nerves, and internal organs. These pressures can easily cause irritation that requires physical adjustment for relief. Overly hard surfaces can cause pain, which will again make you want to move. Sofas and beds with sufficient and well-constructed springs or thick futons placed on the floor usually work quite well. Once you are relaxed enough internally after some lying-down practice has been accomplished, hard surfaces are preferred, because internal relaxation is optimal when there is a strong counterpoint to the body's innate softness. Remember that this practice has been done for millennia on cave floors and in rough mountain hermitages, as well as in comfortable homes with well-designed furniture.

For this style of meditation, you may assume any lying-down position. Most people, however, prefer to lie on the left or right side of the body rather than on belly or back. When lying on your stomach make sure your pillows are arranged in such a way that you have plenty of air. When on your back, place pillows around your head, neck, buttocks, and backs of your knees so you feel no strain whatsoever on your back, neck, or hips.

If you opt for a sideways position, it is best to choose your right side so the weight of your body does not compress your heart and impede the blood circulation. You may cross your left knee over your right knee. If your back or hip is weak or injured, you may want to place a pillow between your knees or around your hips or neck for support. As in the third method of sitting in a chair (see pp. 83–4), it is important for the same reasons to adjust your body in such a way as to lightly stretch, rather than compress, your spinal cord.

How to Practice

Begin every lying-down session by closing your eyes, relaxing your body, and establishing your breathing. Lying down with eyes closed, let go of as much tension as you can, using your awareness to scan internally down from the top of your head to the tips of your toes, progressively releasing all tension you encounter.

Next, still lying down, practice Taoist internal breathing to relax the inside of your body and mind to the maximum extent possible, until eventually the whole inside of your body releases fully. At this juncture, your breathing should have become completely soft, long, deep, and silent. At the point when your breathing becomes so soft it has seemed to disappear, you will, when you breathe, begin to feel a sense of energy coming into your body. Continue breathing until you feel your body filling up with a clean, strong sense of energy from head to toe. It is this vibrant sense of energy that will keep your mind totally awake, even if parts of your body "fall asleep."

Again, this practice is not easy. It usually takes a beginner three to five hours of continuous breathing without moving* to get a complete release without falling asleep. Yet once you have done this practice daily for a few months, you should be able to reach the release point within five minutes, effortlessly. At this point, you are ready to begin the dissolving techniques described in the next chapter.

---

* This amount of practice time must be built up gradually, adhering to the 70% rule to avoid strain.

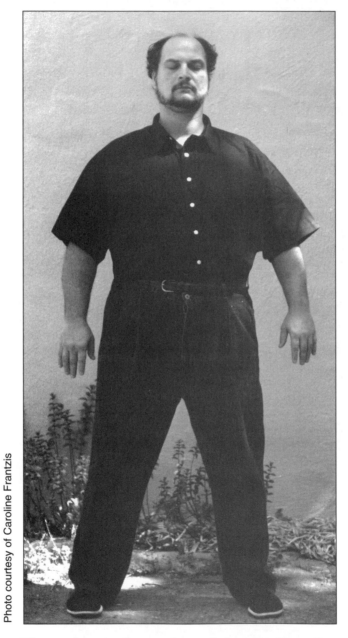

The author is shown here doing the Standing Outer Dissolving process.

The Inner Dissolving Process

CHAPTER
4

I Ching Hexagram 29–Water

If you have integrity
Within your heart lies success
All you do thrives

The Inner Dissolving Process

The Outer Dissolving Process and the Inner Dissolving Process Compared

All the meditation practices of the Taoist water method involve dissolving and resolving the bound blockages of your first six energy bodies until you become internally free. Both the outer and inner dissolving processes begin when you consciously use your awareness to focus your mind on any specific condensed energy shape or pattern within yourself. You then dissipate that shape until it no longer obstructs your mind, body, or spirit in any way. (In all traditions, the conscious use of awareness and attention is a critical basic ingredient to any genuine spiritual meditation method.) You can do each dissolving technique in any one of the five ways–moving, standing, sitting, lying down, or during sexual activity.

The phrase used to describe the outer dissolving process has, for millennia, been "ice to water, water to gas." "Ice" refers to the blocked, congealed energy; "water" refers to the accepting and relaxing of your internal blockage until it no longer causes you tension, while "gas" refers to the *complete release* of all the original bound energy moving away from your physical body. If not completely released, the energy may revert to ice. In contrast, the phrase used for the inner dissolving process of the water method is "ice to water, water to space," where "space" means the vast internal space that exists inside the body, that space being as infinite as the universe.

In the ice-to-water phase of outer dissolving (also used in chi gung and tai chi), the solid, completely bound and condensed energetic shape (ice) is released until it relaxes and reaches the surface of your skin (water). In the inner dissolving process, your bound energy is also released at the point of the blockage until it becomes relaxed, soft, and amorphous (water). Water, however, contains the inherent capacity to recondense to ice. Your "liquid" energy can now move in two different directions: (1) In the outer dissolving process, also used in standing chi gung,* you release your blocked chi from your skin to outside your physical body and then to the edge of your chi/etheric body or even beyond (water to gas). The previously condensed energy is now neutral, unblocked, and shapeless. (2) When you move into the water-to-space phase of the inner dissolving process, on the other hand, you release all blocked content of your *felt* sensations by imploding your energy into the inner space that your previously condensed blocked energy shape occupied, thereby converting your blocked energy into Consciousness without content (a stage of emptiness).

In the early phases of the sitting mode of meditation, it is important that, as you dissolve a blockage, you release its energy inward deeper into your internal space (that is, Consciousness). The Taoist position is that there is as much internal space inside you as there is space in the whole external universe.**

Using the inner dissolving method to go ever deeper inside during sitting meditation, for instance, is like letting your dissolved energy open a door into a door within a door, leading deeper and deeper into inner space in the point at

---

*Chi gung is concerned primarily with physical health, vitality, and the ability to ward off debilitating stress, not with emotional wellness or spiritual enlightenment.

**Over time, in Taoist meditation, the inner and outer dissolving practices are combined, so that as you dissolve inward, either sequentially or simultaneously, you also dissolve outward toward the cosmos. Eventually, this process allows your mind to stabilize in the middle ground, the home of Consciousness, where inner and outer, and that which is neither and both, exist.

which you began dissolving. You implode each layer of energy inward into the point however far it extends internally, until you finally reach a place where your being naturally comes to a stop. This process may proceed very slowly and take long periods of time. Depending on your individual nature, you might experience this endpoint as complete and utter yin or yang energy, a feeling or vision of light, or a sense of water, emptiness, calmness, peace, mind expansion, and so forth. Rest within that endpoint and try to develop the ability to return to that spot through all of the layers of your energy at will and especially in the midst of life's most scary and stressful situations. Eventually, if you dissolve deeply enough into any one spot you will sooner or later end up at your true Consciousness, which, you will discover, has been relieved of the "red dust," or source of your blockage. Consciousness still remains when the red dust goes, and it is at this exact point that you have an experience, whether temporary or permanent, of Consciousness itself.

The Relationship between Mind and Blockage

In the dissolving process, how does your mind contact and then dissolve the tension or blockage in your body, regardless of how dense or subtle that blockage is? In other words, how can you deliberately contact, become aware of and feel the blockages in your body with your mind only? People with normal nerves will feel pain if you hit them forcefully in a sensitive body part. Sometime later, they will feel the "blockages" inside their body as a throbbing pain. Likewise, a person can be erotically stimulated in a sensitive spot and feel pleasure. In strong emotional situations, such as falling in love, experiencing the death of someone close, or being frustrated with situations beyond your control, you can consciously feel your emotions, positive or negative. With a little bit of concentrated "mind effort," you can increase, decrease or mitigate your physical pain, pleasure or emotions. In short, you can indeed feel what happens inside you with your mind.

In externally induced situations, such as those just described, your whole mind, instead of being diffused, concentrates, and all your attention is drawn to the "object" at hand, be it pain, pleasure or emotion. The totality of your awareness, "the subjective observer," is directed at this object. All this requires that the mind be focused, not scattered or distracted. For instance, consider a baby that has fallen down some stairs and has real pain from a physical injury that would normally keep it crying for ten to fifteen minutes. The baby's mind is fully focused on the pain. Every parent knows that if you can distract the baby with something more absorbing than the pain, the baby's attention can be diverted to a new "object," such as a favorite food or a toy. Chances are that the baby will stop crying and focus on the new object. If, in a few minutes, you withdraw the item, the baby will again feel the pain from the fall and will often begin crying anew. Where did the pain from the fall go, and from where did it return? The answer is that the pain went nowhere, the baby's mind did. It takes a certain minimum percentage of your mind's capacity to be consciously aware of anything. In dissolving a blockage, your recognition or interpretation of what you are observing, along with your feelings, is affecting you, the "observer." By going deeper and deeper inside the blockage toward its source, your mind moves further away from the original surface point of contact with the blockage.

Now, how does your mind enter into and resolve the blockage in the first place?

How to Dissolve Inwardly

To an extremely limited extent, a very minimal dissolving of blockages can occur by concentrating our normal *intent* and awareness on them in a relaxed way. For truly effective dissolving to occur, however, both the mind-stream and presence must be involved. *Presence* is a specific felt quality that occurs when all (or almost all) of your aware-ness is fully operational. This presence can be directed at an internal task (such as inner dissolving). When this quality is fully embodied in a person, it naturally exudes outward, affecting others within his or her field; it is this quality that is referred to when we speak of a person "having great presence."

The internal groundwork for recognizing the mind-stream, the motion of the mind, and presence, and for working with these three distinct phenomena, is developed during the preparatory practices. Likewise, the preparatory practices generate the internal mental environment necessary for that "wonderful accident" that allows practitioners direct contact with Universal Consciousness itself. In order to do the beginning outer dissolving practices, which involve only the first two energetic bodies (the physical and the chi), there is no need to recognize the motion of the mind or the mindstream. Again, pure intent will do some small bit of dissolving on its own, but the application of the mindstream and presence is needed for true effectiveness and acceleration of the inner dissolving process.

A critical point for doing all the dissolving practices—especially inner dissolving—is the quality of mind that a practitioner must maintain. Normally in the West when one wishes to concentrate to the utmost, one narrows the focus of his or her mind in a forceful, laserlike manner, which usually creates extreme tension. The inner dissolving practice, in contrast, involves a seeming paradox: you must be continuously highly focused and yet completely relaxed. Your mind releases its strength and opens to maintain the relaxed concentration that lies at the root of Taoist meditation.

This focused yet relaxed state of mind is fundamental and highly valued in both Taoist and Buddhist meditation practices. These two traditions use different metaphors to describe essentially the same point. The Taoists talk about a stone moving through water. The mind is the water: soft, yet capable of moving slowly and calmly or with great turbulence. The stone is the object of your concentration, which the water surrounds. The stone may sink slowly and gradually without obstacle, or be moved up, down, or sideways, depending on the currents that naturally arise.

Shakyamuni Buddha, the story goes, had a talented student who had been a famous musician before devoting his life to meditation. Although he worked immensely hard, the student was not able to penetrate to the depths of his being. When he asked the Buddha what was missing in his practice, the Buddha said he had to tune his mind like a string on his instrument: too loose (too relaxed) and no sound can be made (you might fall asleep), too tight and all you get is a dissonant jangle.

Stage 1. Preparation for Dissolving: Let Your Mind Relax and Settle

In the following pages, the numbered points are instructional, and the bulleted points are suggestions or explanations of more subtle material.

1. Have the *intent* to do the dissolving process. Volitional intent will predispose, rather than directly cause, your mindstream to move toward your blockages.
2. Sit down. It is recommended that the inner dissolving process be done sitting, the outer dissolving process standing.
3. Settle or relax your mind as much as possible.
4. While the mind is settling, your nerves may (and eventually should) begin to relax and your mind should slow down. Your conscious awareness, which is frequently fuzzy or scattered, begins to become more clear and focused. Because your mind or thoughts slow down, the motion of the mind itself begins to slow down, too, thus showing itself more easily and allowing you to recognize or feel a sense of it.
5. Gently focus attention to the act of moving your mind (that is, your conscious awareness) to the top of your head.
6. Wait until your mind begins to move of its own accord to the crown of your head.

7. Once your total mind focuses at the crown of your head, a generalized feeling of the mind expanding, a feeling that is different from your normal state of conscious awareness, should emerge.

8. Feel the sense of the motion of the mind that should now begin to arise.

    • This motion, whether fast or slow, never ceases. It may be smooth and comfortable or rough and at odds with relaxation. Thoughts, ideas, and sensations continuously arise naturally owing to the subliminal content of the mind. Or if there are no discernible thoughts, there is an underlying sense that they are dormant, just below the surface, and sooner or later will manifest as recognizable ideas or feelings.

9. When the ever-growing presence and awareness of the motion of the mind grows sufficiently inside, you become aware of your individual mindstream, which is quite a different thing from the motion of the mind.

    • The mindstream is like the airstream beneath an airplane, which supports the craft in flight, or it can be viewed as the road upon which the motion of the mind rides. The mindstream is the bridge, the connection, between your own ability to be aware and the universal all-pervasive Consciousness itself. The mindstream, as experienced internally, has a particular vibratory feel. It will seem to feel less dense than the motion of the mind and more dense than Consciousness itself.

10. Maintaining your intent at the crown of your head, you now wait until two things happen: your mindstream moves toward the crown of your head of its own accord, and your mindstream and your intent begin to commingle.

Stage 2. The Mindstream Reaches the Blockage

1. Beginning from the crown of your head, or the point at which you want to start the dissolving process (which may be above your head at the boundary of your etheric body), move your awareness downward through your body until you first encounter and feel a blockage.

    •   A blockage is some kind of congealed chi, an uncomfortable or dissonant "something" that is disturbed within the motion of the mind and obstructs some part of it. Blockages can be felt both in the physical body and in the etheric body above your head. If no blockage is present, or if you can't feel one, the motion of the mind will simply continue to move unimpeded.

2. Let your intention to dissolve remain, whether it is subtle or overt.

3. Wait for the mindstream and intention, which are separate, to commingle.

    •   During the rest of the movement toward emptiness and Consciousness itself, the two will remain commingled like the interplay between a singer (your individualized intent) and the band (mindstream). At different times, either may be a little or dramatically louder or softer, both may be equal, or one, although still present, may be virtually inaudible, while the other is loud and completely dominates. Always, however, there will be a flux or flow between your conscious intent, aiding or focusing the ice-water-space process and your felt sense of the mindstream being the primary or sole agent doing the dissolving.

Stage 3. The Mindstream First Enters the Blockage at a Given Point and Begins the Dissolving Process: Ice to Water

At first, the blockage subjectively seems to be something different from you, a foreign object lodged in your awareness but seeming to be some distance from you, even though it is in your mind/body.

1. As your mind moves downward, put your intent on the first place where you feel a sensation of blockage. This is an entry point to the whole blockage but is also a block itself. As the nature of the blockage is holographic, the whole is contained in all of its parts, or points, and all of its points are linked throughout all of your energy bodies. Simultaneously watch the motion of the mind, until the motion of the mind reaches the blockage and you begin to feel it.*

2. Wait actively until you feel your presence grow, and until your mindstream and your intent join. You want your focus and clarity to grow. Do not succumb to the temptation to get drowsy and nod off.

3. Focus your intent on allowing the blocked energy at that point to turn from "ice" to "water."
   - As your presence grows, your awareness of the energetic quality and contours of the block grows along with it.
   - From the beginning, in both the inner and outer dissolving practices, focus on the energy you feel behind (underlying) the blockage more than on the energy of the blockage itself, and on the flow of where the mindstream is going, not just on where it is at any given time.

*The text from here to p. 108 will describe in more detail how, once you can feel the blockage, you dissolve all the way around its perimeter at that height level (stratum), making sure that everything is dissolved–front, back, and sides–before moving on to the next height level of the block, as described in the box "How to Dissolve Downward." on p. 109.

- The growth of your presence further empowers the mindstream to follow your intent and enter the first layer of the blockage at a given point, until the blocked energy there merges with the mindstream, much as an iceberg eventually turns to liquid and merges with the sea.
- The mindstream and your intent become completely commingled. The addition of the mindstream gradually accelerates the inner dissolving process.

Stage 4. The Mindstream Continues Dissolving the First Layer at the Point of Entry of the Blockage: Water to Inner Space

1. Release all the remaining blocked content of your felt sensations by imploding your energy into the inner space that your previously condensed blocked energy shape occupied, thereby converting your blocked energy into Consciousness without content (a stage of emptiness).

2. Let your dissolved energy open a door into a door within a door, leading deeper and deeper into inner space in the point at which you began dissolving. You implode each layer of energy inward into the point however far it extends internally, until you finally reach a place where your being naturally comes to a stop (see p. 97).

    - At this time your intent becomes subordinate to the mindstream, which completely dissipates the energy of the blockage inside your body into inner space, and ideally into emptiness. This process completes the first layer of dissolving your entry point: water to inner space. You may be successful or not–see stage 5.
    - As the releasing of a layer of the point accelerates, the sense of the mindstream can in the beginning (and usually does when you are more experienced)

become clearer and clearer. When a layer of the point where you are holding your awareness fully releases into emptiness, it becomes possible to become aware of the mindstream and the motion of the mind as two clearly differentiated elements connected to your Consciousness, completely separate and yet not intrinsically different, merely different densities of the same parent material.

- Remember that the mindstream is connected to all, not some, parts of your being simultaneously. You can enter into the mindstream from any part of your body, mind, or spirit. There is no true linear sequence of Λ to B to C when releasing layers of a point into inner space.

3. As you move and dissolve into inner space, stay grounded in the background of your awareness by continuously remaining conscious of your entire physical body. *Don't lose a sense of contact with your physical body and go into a purely mental realm.* Continue to dissolve inward into the point at which you entered the blockage, as you simultaneously let yourself experience the dissolving of any associated energies that arise.

- Any blockage located by the inner dissolving process, anywhere in your body, is linked via the mindstream to any other related blockage at any number of points of entry. Any related blockage could be at another point in your physical body or in any of your other energy bodies, and it could either maintain or intensify the effect of the primary blockage. You may temporarily find yourself in such related blockages as you dissolve a layer of the primary blockage. Move with the mindstream but hold some core awareness of the primary blockage as well.
- Some blockages you may encounter will not be extensively linked to other parts of your being;

others may be directly or tangentially linked to thousands of other subsidiary blockages. Some compose core parts of your individual personality or the underlying assumptions and expectations that make up your worldview, that is, how you experience the world you live in.

- Do not confuse the jumping from place to place of the "monkey mind" with the motion of the mind that guides the mindstream to the next linked blockage.

- Your mindstream is like a golden thread simultaneously present in all your energetic bodies, and can, in a microsecond, move between your various energy bodies–from lower to higher and higher to lower. A given energetic blockage could have infinite tributaries (a door within a door within a door) that ultimately lead to a single ocean, where all dissolve. Because of this circumstance and because the motion of mind also has similar properties to the mindstream, your awareness could stay for a considerable time dissolving any specific single place. Or it could skip forward along different tributaries, dissolving and resolving smaller or larger fragments of bound energy, which are directly relevant to the original blockage and must also be resolved in order for the original blockage to be fully released. This movement could be between different energy bodies, causing the practitioner to have successively different internal experiences. As mentioned, all of this can be simultaneously occurring from the one blocked point you are dissolving.

Stage 5. Dissolving All the Successive Layers within a Given Point of Entry and All Other Points at the Same Height of Your Body within a Blockage

1. When you attempt to dissolve a point in a blockage through the first layer of inner space, there are a few possible outcomes:

(a) You are unable to dissolve to a stage of emptiness, and therefore the point of energy is not resolved to a conclusion. Rather, it feels as though it will stay unresolved no matter how long you try to dissolve it. In this case, go to step 2.

(b) You are able to dissolve through the first layer of inner space into a sense of emptiness. You stay in emptiness as long as it lasts. After a while some sense of agitation or additional blocked energy will re-emerge in the same blocked place (which will feel larger than it was, as though you have gone through a door into a larger chamber of your mind). This is a new layer of inner space. The mindstream then follows your intent and the motion of the mind inward again. The mind attempts to dissolve into that layer and resolve it into emptiness. You now dissolve the new larger sense of blocked energy, maintaining the same relationships between motion of the mind, presence, mindstream, intent, and Consciousness itself. If unsuccessful, go to step 2. If successful, wait again for the next layer to arise, and repeat this process.

   • Between the resolution of each layer of the blockage and its next layer will be a resting space where people often feel extremely blissful and at ease with themselves and with creation. This space is where the motion of the mind and the mindstream first make themselves known to your conscious awareness with regularity.

The mindstream and the motion of the mind are usually recognized in one of three forms: specific subtle yet discernible feelings, a level of vibration, or some quality of light.

(c)   After successfully dissolving one or more layers of inner space at a point of entry, you may find, after waiting there, that you sense you have achieved resolution into a final emptiness. Feel whether this resolution has also removed any sense of the blockage. If so, go to step 3. If not, go to step 2.

2.   Transfer any unresolved energy from the original blocked point to the next blocked point at the same height but in front of, behind, or to either side of the original point of entry. If none exists because the blockage has shrunk or moved down, then move down to the next point of entry you can find. Then go back to stage 2 on page 102, and begin again.

- If you try several points of entry and are unable to resolve any to even a first layer of emptiness, then go to step 3 below. If you cannot get access to a blockage, you cannot use its energy to move into emptiness.

3.   With your intent, the motion of the mind, presence, and the mindstream, simply go to the next place down your body where you feel a new blockage and begin all over again.

- Whether you are a beginner or an advanced practitioner, when dissolving (using either the inner or outer process) you move only downward from total blockage to total blockage to ensure that your body's energy channels can handle the energetic load without damage to your central nervous system, that is, damage from whatever energies may be released from your blockages. Dissolving downward is a safety procedure, pure and simple (see Question 10 in Appendix C).

FOCUS ON A SPECIAL TOPIC
How to Dissolve Downward

Consider your body to be a skyscraper of one hundred floors or levels, where your head is the hundredth floor, the soles of your feet the first floor, and the penthouse and basement the etheric body above your head and below your feet. Each floor has, say, fifty rooms on it, some in back, some in front, some on the left side, some on the right. The various blockages that your mind first encounters in the dissolving process are located on specific floors. The rooms are the points of entry.

As your mind stops at a given floor (the hundredth, for example) and steps off the elevator, it may enter one room or several at the same time. When your mind enters one room, let's say Room 130, you begin to dissolve there. When you have completely dissolved whatever is in Room 130, you next mentally go around the building's circumference to all the other rooms on that floor, check if you have other points of entry, and dissolve those wherever you find them. The specific order of rooms you visit on any given floor is random, being determined purely by where your awareness naturally "lands" and finds points of entry into a blockage.

If you cannot dissolve everything in one room and perceive that, no matter how much longer you dissolve, the blockage will not resolve at that point of entry, you next use your intention and awareness to shift whatever energy residue remains in that room to the next room you visit, dissolving any blockages you find in any subsequent rooms on the same floor. You continue this process until the last room on the floor is reached. Either you will dissolve everything on that floor or you will not. Until you get all the way to the bottom of the building, you will continuously alternate between two options:

1.   If your mind does dissolve everything, it gets on the elevator again and starts going down your body, no matter how little or how far, until it encounters the next blocked floor. There you dissolve whatever rooms need it, until you have finished all the rooms on that floor, and your mind goes down to the next blocked floor.

2.   If, however, your mind perceives that it cannot dissolve all the blocked energy in all the rooms on

FOCUS ON A SPECIAL TOPIC
How to Dissolve Downward (continued)

> 2. (cont) that floor, you next take the combined energetic residue from all those rooms and, using your awareness and intention, drop it downward as many or few floors as necessary until your mind encounters another room's felt blockage. There your mind combines the energetic residue from the previous floor with the energy of the new room's blockage, and you dissolve the combined blockage. If successful, you move on until you have dissolved all the rooms on that floor, then go down to the next lower floor. If unsuccessful you drop any energy you cannot dissolve, down to the next lower floor and deposit the energy in the new blockage, combine the energies of the two blockages into one, and do your best to dissolve and resolve the new combined blockage. Next, depending how it goes, you repeat either option 1 or 2.

This description metaphorically shows how the initial stage of the inner and outer dissolving methods work. There is, however, a defining difference between the two methods. With inner dissolving, in a particular room on a particular floor, your mind can find what might be called "chambers" within the room, each one with a door that can lead to what is sensed as a dramatically larger chamber. Your mind locates these chambers when a specific layer of a blockage resolves into emptiness. This path allows your mind to follow the blocked energy to where it is ultimately hiding in your inner space. You pursue it to complete resolution, or if that is not occurring, your mind jumps to another room. In outer dissolving, your mind follows the blocked energy outward, away from the skyscraper (your body) to outer space, past the windows (your skin) into the air around the skyscraper.

Stage 6. Finishing an Inner Dissolving Practice Session

When you realize you are nearing the end of the time you have allotted for practice, take five to ten minutes to do the following steps:

1. Slowly move your intent down your body from the point into which you have been dissolving to your lower tantien.
2. Along the way, take a moment to lightly and quickly dissolve inward at any remaining blockages you may feel.
3. Finally, spend a few minutes dissolving into the lower tantien.

This wrap-up process will help bring energy down your body into your lower tantien, helping center you before stopping. The lower tantien is linked to all points in your physical body. This process will help strengthen those links.

Experiences Often Encountered while Resolving the Successive Layers of a Blockage

In any form of meditation, there is no way to state exactly what experiences an individual will encounter. It would be a mistake to think that "this or that should happen to me," or "I am failing if it does not happen to me." There is simply too much individual variation, which is why teachers are very helpful to sort out your personal specifics from the general points that would be relevant to any individual. Here an attempt is made to indicate what is within normal parameters at progressively more advanced stages.

The ice-to-water and water-to-space stages of inner dissolving should be considered as a continuum rather than two completely separate processes.

Ice-to-Water Stage of the Inner Dissolving Process

1. Feel and observe a blockage.
2. The mindstream contacts the blockage and you have a felt sense of something, possibly a type of vibration or even in relatively rare cases a full-bore vision. Or you start getting various kinds of conceptual ideas, including mental forms or inter-

pretations of what the feelings mean or to what they are specifically connected: for example, physical problems, energetic imbalances or emotional situations involving parents, relationships, anger, depression, or self-image.

3.   Dissolve the initial point of entry. Dissolve through the onion layers of the blockage one by one. How many layers you will eventually go through until a complete resolution occurs, no one can say. What can be said is this:

The cause or causes of the original blockage as you continue dissolving will work their way through each of the energetic permutations that are in some way connected to the blockage. The sense of energy within the mindstream may change, getting stronger, weaker, faster, or slower, but no matter what the change, the underlying "something" (the "form") that allowed you to recognize it in the first place will usually remain until it is dissolved. The subtle quality of the vibration will change to some degree as you move through each stage of emptiness and a new buildup to another resolution.

As you unbind more and more blocked energy and you become involved with the energetic form of the blockage, it is not unusual to begin to spontaneously recognize and interpret emotional and mental meanings related to what you are experiencing while dissolving. This recognition often results in a variety of spontaneously arising insights into the events of your life and the workings of your interior world. When these perceptions occur, it directly indicates that you are working on the third and fourth energetic bodies–the emotional and mental.

Water-to-Space Stage of the Inner Dissolving Process

4.   The overt vibrational form may vanish, leaving
        only a very subtle vibration or only the faintest
        hint of what the blockage means in all its subtle
        aspects. Once the form disappears, over time, its
        charge goes and the form of the blockage seems as
        though it was never there. For example, if you had
        physical pain from a broken bone, the sense of the
        bone itself in that blockage would go away. You
        would be left only with the essence of what the
        broken bone meant to you, in all of its shadings
        and interconnections. If your blockage was
        emotional and related to a situation or person
        (such as a parent, lover, friend, or enemy), the
        sense of the specific situation or person would
        drop away and only the essence of what that
        emotion meant to you would be left. If it was a
        thought, the form of the thought, the specific ideas
        the mind had focused on and recognized, would
        drop, and only the underlying meaning would
        remain when you moved into emptiness. If any of
        these occur, it indicates that you are working on
        your fourth and fifth energetic bodies, the mental
        and psychic.

        From the Taoist perspective, you are now on
        the boundary between secular and spiritual life.
        For most people, going as far as dropping the form
        in the inner dissolving process is more than
        enough to relieve many of life's physical, mental,
        and emotional problems. From this point forward,
        you are now moving into what could be called
        intermediate/advanced spiritual work, which is
        extremely challenging. Up to now, your main
        interest could have been to simply get your inner
        physical, energetic, emotional, and mental life to
        work. From here on, the motivation behind your
        practice must be a sincere interest in spirituality.

5.   Continue dissolving to the next stage of practice. Here the meaning of a blockage and all your interpretations drop. The meaning becomes pure energy without being attached to interpretations or judgments as to what should or should not be. When this process occurs, it indicates that you are working on your fifth energetic (psychic) body. What remains, however, is a clear sense of the self, the "I" that is observing this process.

6.   Now dissolve this sense of self, the "I," until there is only an underlying vibration without a clear sense of any difference between the vibration and yourself. Dissolving the sense of the "I" is not easy and requires a great deal of sensitivity and relaxed focus. At this level, the volume of subtle distractions that take you away from dissolving seems to expand exponentially. Working at this level does not mean you are transcending your "ego"; however, it is a definite step in the right direction. Taoist meditators consider the dropping of the "I" to be the true beginning of entering the final stage of moving into the personal connection to Consciousness itself.

     At this point, it is not unusual for you to start experiencing some level of inner light–not a light you purposely visualize but one that spontaneously arises when enough obstacles are removed between your normal awareness and Universal Consciousness. When this experience occurs, it indicates that you are beginning to work on your sixth (causal) energetic body. What remains, however, is the underlying core of the blockage.

7.   In this next plateau, you dissolve the underlying subtle vibration or sense of light that remains after the sense of the gross "I" drops away. This sense will be very clear, and it will be a real challenge to dissolve it into emptiness. At this juncture, the

veils between where you are and the full resolution of the blockage will come, one after another,
each one being more subtle and difficult to
dissolve than the one before. When this situation
occurs, it indicates that you are working further
into your sixth (causal) energetic body.

8.   You have now achieved a complete sense of emptiness, and your inner world is becoming more and
more still. The next plateau is exceptionally difficult. It usually takes some time before your sensitivity can adjust sufficiently to working with it
well. There are myriad energetic veils between the
initial sense of emptiness and Consciousness, each
more subtle than the last. As you clear out the veils
one by one, you begin to get glimpses of
Consciousness. It is as though there is a light bulb
with hundreds of layers of gossamer over it. When
enough layers disappear, even if just for a second,
you see some light, no matter how obscured. As
more veils fall away, as more of your internal
content loses its charge, you view Consciousness
through fewer and fewer filters.

Eventually your mind becomes yet more still
and you start experiencing Consciousness in a
"now you see it, now you don't" fashion. In the
beginning, you glimpse a little, then wait a long
time for the next peek. Gradually, the gaps shorten
and you become increasingly familiar with
Consciousness. When you gain the awareness, it
indicates that you are working yet more deeply
into your sixth (causal) energetic body and are on
the border between the sixth body and the seventh
(the body of individuality).

9.   In the next phase, your mind finally becomes still
and the barriers between your normal awareness
and Consciousness dissolve away in every single
blockage simultaneously, as you enter into the
Great   Stillness.   You   become   aware   of

Consciousness as a living entity that becomes a lifelong companion. Meditation must be continued, however, or more "red dust" will collect, again creating veils that have to be dissolved in order for you to be aware of Consciousness effortlessly and at all times. You have now moved into the seventh body and are ready to begin working with it.

An individual who has come this far–to the Great Stillness–has completed the intermediate stage of Taoist meditation and is prepared to learn inner alchemy.

What Might Happen along the Way

As you dissolve and encounter different energetic bodies, you experience the energy in the blockage growing, completing, and dropping. The Taoists call these energetic phenomena the "ten thousand experiences." It is impossible to say what specific experiences any individual may or may not have. It is also very difficult to describe in words the real qualities of these experiences, which can be quite different from those we encounter in normal life, read about in poetry, or obtain from a hypnotic induction.

The important point to remember is that the experiences themselves are not significant or required for progress. They merely may or may not happen, and having specific experiences does not make you better or worse; it only means that something happened to you and not someone else. Only a small percentage of meditation experiences convey useful information that indicates the need to expend energy in further investigation.

There are vibrations or qualities of light that mimic the underlying tones and shadings of various sections of our interior world. These vibrations create the subliminal energetic foundations upon which we experience life. The difference is that they are more distilled and lie at the very heart of how and why we all act in the world and experience our inner selves. You may experience light or vibration localized at the point you are dissolving, throughout your whole body, or even outside your body; or you may feel it in one tantien, in two or all three tantiens at once, or in any combination of energy channels.

The vibrations may range in impression from mildly pleasant to almost blissfully orgasmic, from merely normal to downright odd, or from mildly irritating to disturbing beyond belief, seemingly the essence of frustration (or anger, depression, loneliness, anxiety). The vibrations can be very much of this world or extremely otherworldly, both ethereal and dark. They can lull you into drowsiness or shock you into being exceptionally awake. The vibrations can induce you to feel wary or completely trusting. They can be experienced as almost anything that is within the scope of human possibility to feel and imagine.

Light may be experienced as a cool ocean breeze on a beautiful tropical beach or as cold emanating from the deepest reaches of outer space; it may be as warm as the blue waters of the Caribbean, as hot as a boiling cauldron, or searing with a laser-like quality that obliterates all in its path. Light may appear as if it were solid or without substance, or it may have various intensities, from white light to all the colors of the rainbow. The light may appear as lightning, pulses, or star dust.

You may feel either vibration or light as being as dense and compressed as a black hole or as expanding and bright as the subatomic particles released by an exploding sun. In short, almost anything, including formlessness yet with form, and emptiness pregnant with possibility.

Ideas may be floating in your head, both within and quite beyond the realm of normal imagination. All kinds of ideas–creative, mundane, orthodox, joyous, painful, the deepest and darkest ever, what you expect, or beyond what you ever considered possible. Sooner or later, however, regardless of the idea you have, its opposite is bound to occur: physical sensations of immense sensitivity, many beyond normal conception; trancelike experiences as well as those of complete lucidity; gross as well as extremely refined emotions and psychic experiences; feelings of being and of nonbeing, of being corporeal and without a body. All, some, a little, or none of these feelings may happen to you, and then again, they may not. All that can be said is that whatever energies you experience, you will sooner or later also experience their opposites.

Outer and Inner Dissolving Compared for Ease of Practice

Although both the outer and the inner dissolving processes are part of the same circle, the inner dissolving process is initially more difficult to do than the outer dissolving process for several reasons:

1.   The first phase of the outer dissolving process initially works with only the first two energy bodies, the physical and energetic. The inner dissolving process works with the first seven energy bodies, a more complex task.

2.   The outer dissolving process does not require you to have a sense of the motion of the mind or the mindstream. The process does, however, create an environment in which the practitioner gains practical experience of the normal motion of the mind first and the significantly more subtle mindstream later. Whether or not a practitioner is deliberately looking for mind and mindstream, they will be found. The outer dissolving process, along with the other preparatory practices, also usually creates "the wonderful accident" in which you can spontaneously encounter Consciousness itself.

In the inner dissolving process you can work through the first two energy bodies and, to a limited extent, the emotional body without any need to experience the subtleties of the motion of the mind and the mindstream. To move into the higher energy bodies, however, it helps to have personal contact with the motion of the mind and the mindstream. It also helps to have had the "wonderful accident" through the outer dissolving process so that when you move toward Consciousness you recognize your experiences rather than ignore and deny them, either through ignorance or skepticism.

3.   Initially, the outer dissolving process provides the key to unlock the door behind which lies the world of inner dissolving. Conversely, the inner dissolving process provides the motion of the mind and the mindstream, which is the key to unlocking the door to the higher bodies using both the inner and outer dissolving processes simultaneously. This interplay conforms to a basic operational principle of Taoist meditation: "There is as much inside as there is outside, and as much outside as there is inside."

4.   The imploding and exploding of the two dissolving processes have aspects that are intrinsically different. Most societies are externally oriented. Western society for the past several hundred years has employed much of its energies outwardly in gaining dominion over the earth. Because of this inclination, Western minds are geared to thinking externally. If we can see or feel something externally, we usually have the possibility of at least imagining it in some context. Our culture reinforces the need to develop our external senses: touch, seeing, hearing, tasting, and smelling. There is not much in Western culture that values developing our inner senses or even "believing" they exist. Most people in the West consider it strange to have inner senses, something many ancient civilizations and prescientific cultures considered a natural human birthright.

The inner senses allow a person to directly perceive the chi of something, rather than just its external manifestation. If you have natural psychic sensitivity, it is often easier to feel energy outside your body than to feel the energy within it. Even for authentic psychics, it is often a more difficult task to feel energy inside the body. However, because you can see things outside your body and can feel the space outside your body by moving your hand through it, you have the possibility of imagining energy there and ultimately becoming able to actually sense it. It is also relatively easy to focus on relaxing soft tissues and deeper substructures inside the body, because you have physical nerves there. For the inner dissolving process to go far into a micro-dot of space, you have to develop not merely your physical nerves but also an inner sense of the significantly more subtle energy channels and the Consciousness inside your body.

The End Result of the Dissolving Process

The end stage of the dissolving process involves more advanced levels of meditation. The more experience you have with meditation, the easier it will be to comprehend its full value. Taoism, Buddhism, and the Hindu yogic traditions more or less share this same methodology of working with Consciousness. This is the way in which samadhi or "absorption into the absolute" is accomplished in yoga. In like manner, the water-to-space concept is used in Taoism. The observer "I" focuses its attention either on a physical object, whether outside or inside the body, or on a mental, emotional, physical, or psychic phenomenon, or a feeling, ghost, or image. From the interaction between the observer (subjective viewer/seer) and the observed (object/blockage), meanings or interpretations arise. These often become more refined. Each interpretation can yield up a more expanded realization of the interconnections between your object and everything that is tangential to it, no matter how slightly, until finally, in your mind, the meanings drop away. Even the object "dissolves" (or, in yogic language, becomes absorbed) until you go from water to inner space and everything becomes empty. At this point, your awareness is flowing steadily toward the object in an unbroken, nondistracted fashion so that the energy of the object unravels and breaks up and you become cognizant of what has occurred. As this disintegration happens, any attachments you have to the object also break up so that you resolve and embrace all the meanings of the object. The freed energy converts to spirit as you begin to move from water to inner space.*

Then the meaning "drops" or "dissolves," and only you, the observer, remains. As you keep on dissolving, the sense of "I," the observer, drops or dissolves, and you attain an inward stillness in which neither the form of the object, its meaning, nor a sense of yourself impinges on your complete awareness of Consciousness itself. Prior to this, you have ignored your Consciousness (as happens when you are internally blocked or cut off). Or you have been completely absorbed with some aspect of the content attached to your Consciousness–the object's external form, meaning, interpretation, or sense of self. Each state of stripping this content increases the mind's "emptiness of content."

When you dissolve your content, two things happen: (1) the emotional and psychic forces inside you become resolved, and (2) the hidden and beneficial qualities of Consciousness itself are released so that they permeate the entire structure of your being, as opposed to merely causing a fleeting experience. Something inside you shifts and stays, never to go back. To whatever depth you have penetrated your physical or "psychic knot" (yogic terminology), when you have reached absorption (fully dissolved and relaxed it), you will gain "knowledge of it" (yogic terminology). This knowledge will naturally bring insights into that object, such

---

*See the section "Jing (Body), Chi (Energy), Shen (Spirit)" in Chapter 2 of *Relaxing into Your Being*.

as its intrinsic nature, where it comes from, the mechanisms of how it interacts and changes under various conditions and stimuli. Ultimately, at the successful conclusion of the samadhi/absorption or ice-to-space process, you achieve freedom from all the energetic and psychic attachments that bind and torture your body, mind, and soul/consciousness. With that freedom comes a release that allows your body, mind, and Consciousness to be totally at ease and comfortable, imbued with a spontaneously arising natural sense of inner stillness, quiet, peace, and joy.

Whole Mind Concentration and Distraction

In order to move into this relaxation, and into the natural state of your Consciousness, there are two barriers to be overcome. The first is how to maintain the continuous focus of your "whole mind's" concentration (presence), and the second is how to deal with the problem of distraction. It helps to look at the body/mind as being simultaneously both an interconnected web of sequential cause and effect and a hologram in which anything that is happening in one part is instantaneously communicated to every other part with no time lag. The "water to inner space" phase and the moving into emptiness are related to the instantaneous hologram effect, whereas the "ice to water to almost space" is related to the sequential web.

The first difficult problem is getting the mind to be able to focus on an object in a continuous, unbroken stream. The easiest objects for the mind to feel and focus on are the physical body and the energy that makes the body work: the chi. Much harder are the emotions (emotional body). Harder still are ideas (mental body), and the hardest objects to keep focusing on are psychic and causal energies (psychic and causal bodies). A few rare individuals come by this ability to concentrate naturally. Most of us, though, do not, and neither have we undergone any systematic training that would allow conscious thought to focus on such subtleties without becoming easily distracted.

The ability to hold the concentration steady, in a relaxed fashion, requires the use of the whole mind. Traumas, dead spots, or internal conflicts are "stored" in the body as blockages, and their energies, as you stir them up, can render you incapable of achieving a relaxed, whole-mind concentration. The less of your mind you can use, the less ability you have to remain consciously focused on an object of your intentions. This procedure requires a relaxed strength of mind. The strength of mind to concentrate on an object (internal or external) can be likened to the strength needed to lift a weight. To be able to focus your mind on your hand may require ten units of strength; to focus on your chi, one hundred units; emotions, one thousand; mental, ten thousand; psychic, one hundred thousand; and causal, one million. As a first step, your mindstream must have the strength to "lock onto" an object with continuous concentration.

The preparatory practices of Taoism (chi gung, internal martial arts, Taoist yoga, etc.) begin the metaphorical weight-lifting that progressively develops your concentration through repetition and habit. Each time you practice, mental strength (that is, the percentage of your mind devoted to the concentration) increases. Many people's minds are simply fragmented, with many things going on at the same time. This weakens their capacity to pay attention to one thing to the exclusion of all others for a set period of time. In Zen, this ability is called one-pointed concentration. In sports and science it is called focus. Successful people usually have focus and mediocre people usually do not. A major purpose of all classical education from ancient Greece to today was to develop a mind that had the capacity to concentrate and reflect.

Now, as mentioned, for you to continuously focus on your physical body or chi body is a relatively easy task compared to an attempt to focus on your higher bodies. There are two ways the mind contacts an object. The first is that we see it, touch it, hear it, and recognize it, with the middle ground between the object and the mind not being in our conscious awareness. The second way is for the mind to be conscious of its own mindstream, which is attached to the mind, and both of them together make a tangible connection to the object. If this mindstream is kept continuous, it can "lock onto" the object and, by increasing its power, enter the object. The preparatory practices can develop the mind-stream's strength to the point where it is capable of continuous focus on the body, chi, and the initial contact with the emotional energy of the body. Inner dissolving can ultimately develop the midstream's strength to a true whole-mind state of 100 percent concentration, free from distraction.

Dealing with Distraction

While you develop a relaxed strength of mind, you must also look out for another obstacle in meditation–distraction. When a person puts his or her focused attention on an internal or external object, a common process occurs in stages. Initially, attention is continuous and clear; then you become distracted and lose focused attention. If you return to concentration with a sense of being spaced out or disoriented, you will know that distraction has taken place. If, however, you return to concentration with attention more or less on the object, you may not be aware of having blanked out at all. Sometimes, when you come back to focus, you are able with renewed vigor to resume your focus from where it left off before the distraction. At other times, however, you may have a sense of unease and disquiet that will not let you continue your concentration. Often, your internal dialogues or subliminal mental images predominate, and you are not able to continue. Or your focus may be evenly divided between the object of your concentration and tangential internal happenings of which you may or may not be consciously aware. Questions arise from this situation: What happens internally when you get distracted? What is the internal mechanism of the distraction process? How can it be overcome?

The process goes like this: You are meditating–you become distracted–you focus again for a shorter or longer duration–you get distracted and go blank again–you focus again–you become half focused, half distracted–you become totally distracted and blank out–you return, and so forth. What happens when the mindstream goes totally blank or becomes partially distracted? What is the nature of the black hole our conscious awareness falls into?

When we encounter a situation that is painful or over-whelming, or that challenges our very sense of sanity or internal tolerance to stress or the unknown, we often cannot fully experience that situation for what it is. Something in us disconnects from the event, to give us enough internal distance to avoid its intensity. Some of us go totally numb inside, some partially numb, just to avoid dealing with the event. Take, for example, rejection in romantic love. Those who have suffered this rejection often carry their pain over to their subsequent love relationships by withdrawing into a black hole of internal distraction whenever they start to be fully engaged with another.

Many people, when they experience a traumatic or overwhelming event in their lives, find they can't quite remember what happened for hours, days, weeks, months, or years. That whole period of time seems a blank, a limbo. The sense of this drift itself ultimately must be dissolved if the meditator is to connect the gaps between one conscious awareness and another. In meditation this blank drifting space can go on for hours on end without abatement or can occur ten times, in micro-units, within a few seconds.

Resolving these "distraction gaps" happens both by focusing on the obvious content that naturally arises in your mind (that is, on what happened to cause the distraction) and by dissolving the formless gaps, those places where you just drift. You dissolve disconnected dead spots within yourself that are just as real and as much a piece of your mindstream's content as any physical, energetic, emotional, mental, or psychic pain or pleasure.

It may appear to you that nothing is happening when in reality you are ridding yourself of a major structural part of every beginning meditator's interior landscape. Each time you practice by releasing some of the energy of the "dead spot," your relaxed ability to be continuously aware of your mindstream gets stronger and stronger. When the work gets boring–"nothing is happening"–you are often in truth connecting up the distracted gaps in the web of your consciousness. Many of these gaps come from the time when we were in the womb and could not handle all the sensations and input coming into us from our mother. The overwhelming flood of sensations we were not capable of dealing with then created a structural "distracting fog" in our consciousness, which we would use for the rest of our life to avoid dealing with life's problems. As a result, we often miss experiencing life's finest joys.

Working through these "fog gaps" and dissolving them gradually enables us to get to the real energetic blockages that bind us–in Chinese terminology, our ghosts. Dissolving the fog sets the stage for releasing the ghosts. So when you reach a "fog" point, keep dissolving that point until you arrive at what is behind it.

The dissolving process then proceeds: Dissolve the sensation of the blockage–dissolve the fog–return to the blockage again–dissolve the fog–reach down to the end of the content–release all the fog holding internal content–remain on the content until it all releases–dissolve until it becomes empty and still–dissolve the emptiness and any fog commingled with it until you completely internally relax where the blockage once was. Stay in this comfortable, relaxed state until it reintegrates back into your mindstream without tension and your physical body becomes relaxed, vibrant, calm, and comfortable with itself.

Much of the inherent tension and malaise within us is caused both by the conflicts of the "ghosts" contained in blockages and by the "fog" that keeps us like zombies, neither fully alive nor completely dead. The water method of Taoist meditation overcomes both through the dissolving process. As you begin meditating, the distractions prevail over continuous awareness. This reverses over time. In the final stages, as your experience of your mindstream strengthens, it becomes as important to be as aware from each micro-second to micro-second as you previously were from hour to hour. When your mindstream no longer becomes distracted, you will be able to be internally still and aware of Consciousness itself. Then you are ready to transmute the emanating quality of your Consciousness, and ready for internal alchemy.

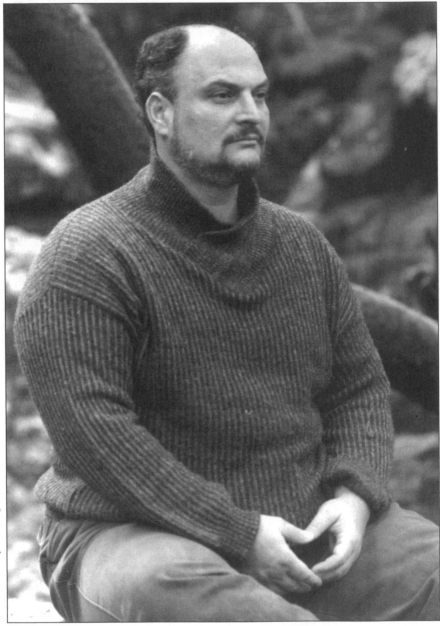

The author is shown here doing the Inner Dissolving process.

Dissolving Blockages in Your Physical, Chi, and Emotional Bodies

CHAPTER
5

I Ching Hexagram 24–Return

On the seventh day comes return
It benefits to move in a clear direction

Dissolving Blockages in Your Physical, Chi, and Emotional Bodies

When you systematically use the dissolving practices, there is a generally recommended progression–first you focus on the physical body, then the chi (etheric) body,* and then the emotional body.** With the physical body, you begin your dissolving at the top of your head and over time–and probably many practice sessions–dissolve until you have cleared your body of blockages of a physical nature all the way to the bottom of your feet. Then you move on to focusing on blockages in the chi body, where you begin dissolving at the top of your etheric body above your head and dissolve down, finishing at your lower tantien (see Appendix D). You then start again above the head and dissolve down to the bottom of your etheric body below your feet. Then you might take on the emotional body, where you follow the same progression as for the etheric body–from the top of the etheric body to the lower tantien and then from the top to the bottom of the etheric body. Your work on any one of these stages might take months or even years to accomplish. After you have repeatedly practiced dissolving blockages in each

*For definitions of the chi body and etheric body refer to *Relaxing into Your Being,* pp. 51-2.

**Procedures for dissolving blockages in the other five energy bodies exist but are outside the scope of this volume.

of the three bodies separately and are beginning to feel and recognize the different qualities of their energies, you may begin, during a single pass from top to bottom, to work on whatever comes up from any of these bodies.

Dissolving Blockages in Your Physical Body

An experience from your past (an injury or sickness, for example) may become lodged in a particular place in your physical body. When you encounter such a blockage, focus your mind on gently dissolving whatever it is. Use your mind to modify the vibratory frequency of the blockage until it breaks up. In the process of dissolving a given block, you may well experience to some degree whatever is stored inside that block. For example, suppose you want to heal an old injury or increase blood flow in previously traumatized blood vessels brought about by, say, a sports accident or surgery or disease. As you release the bound energy of that given spot (the remnants of the old sports injury), you may actually feel the same physical pain (or a shadow-like variation of it) that came with the original mishap.

Dissolving blockages in your physical body will increase all aspects of your physical ability, including your speed, strength, balance, and general health. The Chinese use Taoist meditation to improve overall circulation, target blood movement to specific spots within the body, and heal illnesses or injuries. In Chinese medicine, most, if not all, diseases are viewed as caused by blockages of chi or blood in the body.

Dissolving Blockages in Your Chi Body

At the next level of practice, you will systematically work with and dissolve the components of your chi body, the first of your subtle energy bodies. The chi energy referred to here is that which runs through the thousands of energy lines that make your body a living thing, more than just a fleshly bag of water and chemicals. The physical body and the more subtle chi that runs through it are difficult to separate at first. If you keep your mind focused and work slowly and softly, however, the differences will sooner or later become clear.

You will want eventually to dissolve all the components of the various major physical and energetic systems inside your body, including your energy gates; right, left, and central channels; all acupuncture meridians (and critical acupuncture points, when appropriate); small secondary energy linkages; internal organs; glands; and the three tantiens. When working with the even more subtle sensations of your chi body (instead of only your physical body), you follow the same procedures as when dissolving the physical body.

At every level of practicing Taoist meditation, you may be flooded with sensations. Do not place too much emphasis on them, for they pass like ever-changing clouds in the sky. Generally, most are unimportant; only a tiny percentage actually indicate something clearly needing resolution. Simply go through each sensation as it arises and carefully dissolve it inward or outward or both, in order to be free from it. As you go through each sensation, it will probably be replaced by yet another one. Think of the process as detective work, where you act upon one clue at a time until you reach the source of all the sensations.

For example, a specific area of your body may have a general overall sensation of, say, lightness. Yet in the midst of the lightness is a place that feels heavy and broken up. What you are feeling may be a physical abnormality of some sort, perhaps a constricted blood vessel or scarring retained from an injury. Or if the sensation is an intermittent heavy/light spiking phenomenon, it may be a malfunctioning acupuncture meridian. Or the heaviness might be emotionally based. It could, for instance, represent one of the following:

- An emotional trauma locked into your body (divorce, death of someone close, disappointment, failure).

- An unexpressed or overexpressed emotion (anger, fear, depression, lust, insecurity, pride) that has become lodged in your body from a past event and recurs as a habit bearing little relation to the events in your current life.
- A mental block that binds intellectual or psychic capacities that are hidden in your consciousness waiting to be awakened.

Individuals feel things in their own unique styles, and two persons may have widely divergent causes for what appear to be similar sensations. For that reason it is impractical to attempt to analyze the causes of specific body sensations in a short description of meditation.

From the point of view of Taoism, the dissolving of the physical and chi bodies merely sets the stage for a person to begin the process of spiritual evolution, which is about finding that mysterious something that is changeless throughout all time, space, and circumstances, rather than the physical body, which normally is a temporary phenomenon. Before continuing on the path of meditation, you need to ask yourself if you are honestly willing to accept the responsibilities of an inner spiritual life, which will most likely be more challenging than remaining oblivious to your spirit and remaining connected only to the details of the external world.

Dissolving Blockages in Your Emotional Body

After you have released whatever bound energy you can feel in your physical and chi bodies, you can then begin to work with your emotional body to release the emotional trauma that is bound there. Unless you have lived your entire life in unusually benevolent circumstances, you have experienced emotional trauma at some point in your life. Whether the traumas are major or minor, the results do not differ appreciably in that both destroy some portion of your peace of mind. The nature of emotional suppression is such that when you receive powerful emotional shocks, your conscious mind may not remember how deeply it affected you, or even that it influenced you at all. Nevertheless, the shocks are still there.

The Taoist point of view, accepted increasingly in the West, is that your emotions are literally stored within your body.* Within your physical tissue are the energies of numerous energetic bodies, including your chi and emotional bodies. These vibrate at higher frequencies of subtle energy than your physical body. This form of storage is possible because all eight bodies exist at the same time and place at different vibratory frequencies in a given physical form and consciousness.

When you first learn to dissolve emotional energy, it is best to use the inner dissolving method because it is more effective than the outer dissolving method. Within your capacity to do so, you want to dissolve the bound energy of stuck emotional traumas in the same way that you dissolve the bound energy in your physical and chi bodies. Begin the inner dissolving process by starting at the boundary of your etheric (chi) body outside your physical body and moving down and inward through your physical body. As you meditate, put your attention on whatever emotions naturally come up. In this manner, you can unravel your emotional traumas.

Past traumas continue to exert a disruptive influence in the present in part because when we experience a traumatic event, most of us never sufficiently express our emotions *at the time the trauma occurs*. As we grow from child to adult, we are all subjected to societal rules, both written and unwritten, that constrain the way that we can react emotionally. Consequently, the suppression of emotion is a

---

*The growing field of psychoneuroimmunology demonstrates how the body secretes substances that directly induce mental and emotional states and how, in turn, those states directly affect physiological functions. Within the discipline of psychology, body-centered schools of psychotherapeutic technique are also gaining more acceptance. After deep tissue massage (physical) or acupuncture therapy (energetic)—each form of therapy in general having no inherent psychological element—individuals will often find themselves spontaneously experiencing emotional mood swings or releases, both quiet and cathartic.

very common behavior. The result is that we have stored our pain or rage or frustration or confusion. We pay for such suppression with ever-increasing emotional dysfunction and upheaval and the inability to enjoy the present moment fully or deal responsibly with important issues in our lives because of unconscious denial. The blocked emotional energies remain stored in our bodies, inhibiting the full expression of our emotions in the present.

Taoists are quite familiar with suppressed emotional trauma and place great importance on releasing it. After all, these Taoist practices originated in imperial China, where expressing how you really felt about something before the all-powerful aristocracy and bureaucracy could have resulted in immediate torture or death, for yourself and your family. In their own way, many modern politically free societies are also repressive, although their behavioral controls are more or less covert. Taoist meditation allows you to quietly release the deep-seated emotional traumas stemming from the stress of contemporary living without letting others know what you are doing. It is vitally important to remove them, for emotional traumas often cause internal hesitations that inhibit or stop our ability to change.

As mentioned, when you are traumatized or emotionally attacked, the energy of the event can freeze deep inside your body and grow. You might think of the process as a grain of sand irritating an oyster and growing into a pearl (which bears no outer resemblance to a grain of sand) as the oyster tries to suppress the irritation. However, what grows inside us is not a beautiful pearl but something ugly.

Three Methods for Releasing the Emotions

Method 1. Dissolving without an Agenda

The first method of releasing the bound energy of emotional traumas through Taoist meditation is begun by sitting and taking note of whatever happens to come to mind. Do not try to resolve or analyze it. Slowly and gently move the energy of your body and mind in the general direction of where your mind is being drawn. At this point, you can begin to use the same procedure you used to dissolve bound energy in your physical and chi bodies–that is, start at the top of the chi body above the head and move your awareness carefully and slowly downward through your chi body and to your physical body. As you move from above your head downward, you may get a sense of energy or emotion in a place in your chi or physical body. Remain at that point and dissolve it to the extent you are able, using the inner dissolving techniques described in the previous chapter.

Concentrate on the energy of the emotion itself and the energy that is lurking behind it, and not on any conscious thoughts you may have about it. The conscious thinking may be a smoke screen. As you dissolve the layers of bound emotional energy in a particular place, you may eventually have some kind of inner release and reach some sort of peace with it. If this resolution happens, either at once or after a while, you may have a peaceful respite. If the blockage is not fully resolved, other dissonant feelings, thoughts, or energies will sooner or later naturally begin to arise. Again, you may or may not consciously comprehend them. Concentrate on the sensation of energy underlying your conscious thoughts, the subtle energetic sensation that is generating those thoughts or emotions, rather than the conscious thoughts themselves. If you can, be aware of the more subtle energy or sensation felt just behind the obvious one you are working with. This same procedure is followed in both inner and outer dissolving practices.

Try not to get distracted. If you do, dissolve the "fog" and then the energy source again. As you go through your blockage layer by layer, like peeling an onion, you will find and dissolve traumas that are deeper and deeper inside you.

Fully experience the energies moving anywhere in your body. Do not fight them or hold them back, but at the same time don't get caught up in them. Allow as much as possible of the releasing energy to help carry you inward; let the remaining energies course through and out of your body.

Sometimes you will consciously recollect or re-experience past trauma. However, you are more likely to feel or experience emotions or energies that have no obvious connection to each other or to the factual source of your trauma. These "facts" may not be necessary or useful to know. Releasing emotional energy can create an even greater flood of sensations than dissolving physical or chi blockages. Trauma can create energy waves in your system that have no recognizable shape. It is not functionally important to understand intellectually what is going on: *it is important to release the block*. As you release more and more of this trapped energy, things will leave you, although you may have no idea what they were.

As the internal pressure repeatedly builds and subsides, you may become aware of even more subtle emotions that had been denied or ignored, consciously or unconsciously. When you reach the end of one emotional trauma, there are many others to work on. It is therefore somewhat useless to become attached to or proud of the work you have done, as such attachment wastes time and energy that can be more profitably applied to resolving other emotional suppressions.

Method 2. Dissolving with an Agenda

If you are aware of a particular trauma or a specific event that you need to release, you can work from the beginning specifically on that bound energy. Instead of lightly flowing into whatever trauma randomly comes to mind, you can gently hold this trauma or life-sapping emotional pattern with your conscious awareness for the entire meditation session as you dissolve its energy. As in Method 1, let the energy of the trauma or pattern arise, start at the top of your chi body, and begin to dissolve at the first blockage of any kind you find on the way down.

Often, if you ponder a specific trauma or pattern before you meditate, you predispose your mind in that direction, and you will almost automatically fall into working with that emotional trauma or pattern. If not, simply dissolve whatever naturally arises. Frequently, seemingly trivial side issues resolve the big issue. Therefore, make no attempt to control the specifics of how the meditation develops, but follow the natural flow of internal events that your general intention is spontaneously bringing up.

Suppressed emotions can diminish your vitality. However, you can also express your emotions *too much*. Such overexpression or continuous catharsis can cause ongoing irritation of your emotions, so that the more they are violently expressed, the more they want to explode or take all your energy away from you. Fortunately, dissolving works on both underexpression and overexpression of emotions. Remember that emotions provide the spice in life (one does not want to use meditation to become an unfeeling robot), but emotions can be a problem when they become unbalanced. They can destroy a human being from the inside out.

Method 3. Using the Shocks of Life

Life sometimes brings sudden instantaneous shocks that can come out of nowhere. These can be of any kind–physical, financial, emotional, political, natural (physical disasters), or against your reputation. For example, your life is running smoothly until one day your body is smashed in a freak accident, your whole savings are lost in a stock market crash, a loved one becomes deathly ill, or you are framed and arrested for murder. Such events send tremendous shocks of energy through your system.

Often, the energy from shock becomes buried deep in the mind and is held there for a long time after the initial trauma has occurred. Some individuals undergo counseling or therapy for months or years to resolve the aftermath of a great shock. It is, then, helpful to understand the energetic nature of a shock to the system.

When a strong shock comes your way, its energy enters your body and mind. When it first enters, you tremble and are frequently so overwhelmed that you do not realize its full impact. At this point, the effect of the shock is relatively easy to dissolve, resolve, and release with the inner dissolving practice. After the energy of the shock hits you, it initiates a strongly felt or subliminal wave that moves through your first six energy bodies. This wave then activates all the hidden and repressed inner contents of your consciousness that have similar energetic shapes or vibratory configurations. The activating and supercharging of all these other shapes is often more destabilizing than the initial shock itself.

These shocks, which are normally considered "bad things," are perceived in Taoist thinking as meditation gifts from the gods. How can a painful, stressful event be a gift? The answer is that if, soon after the shock, you engage and dissolve the immediate trauma, and then use that energy to keep dissolving deeper, you may gain easy and rapid access to many other hidden and suppressed energy blockages that have been shaken loose by the original shock. This dissolving practice can be the most intense of the three methods. It can dramatically accelerate your ability to clear out the internal garbage of your personal emotional and psychic basement. This third method of resolving shocks back to their source and much further beyond has the capacity to free an individual for life from powerfully entrenched emotional, mental, and psychic obstacles. Both major and minor discomforts of the body and mind that would ordinarily take years of generalized meditation to resolve can sometimes be cleared up for good in a matter of days, weeks, or months using this method.

The Emotional Dissolving Technique and Its Implications for Astrology

Although clearing your physical, chi, and emotional bodies can take years to accomplish, you must recognize that these are only the most elementary of the Taoist meditation

FOCUS ON A SPECIAL TOPIC
Dissolving Shock

One of my students was at Candlestick Park in San Francisco watching the 1989 World Series when a major earthquake struck. He witnessed the entire baseball stadium shake and the concrete walls undulate directly behind his seat. This was a powerful event that severely affected him, as it did many others in the Bay Area. He came to class hours later, visibly shaken. He had clearly experienced severe emotional trauma. His complexion, normally dark, was now ashen gray, the blood having drained from his face. He was clearly deeply upset. Earthquakes release an incredible energy wave that vibrates both the gross and subtle aspects of anyone's being.

This student began practicing dissolving at once. Because he dealt with the energetic trauma immediately, he was able to disperse it before it settled in his body. He was also able to use the shock of the earthquake to access and dissolve other long-held emotional blockages in his system, even those back to his childhood that he had been previously unable to access or resolve. It took days, but he was able to use the shock to his advantage. Shortly afterward he had no emotional residue from the earthquake. Many others in the Bay Area were not so fortunate. The longer the time you wait from the source of the shock, the harder it is to dissolve and resolve its residue.

practices. Later you start to work with your other five energy bodies and the energy outside your body. The Taoists found that what happens inside you correlates directly with the universe outside your physical body. For example, your chi body is larger than your physical body. As you clear your chi by going inside, you can also clear your chi on the outside, as it extends outside your physical form from just a few feet to over one hundred feet. When the chi is bound inside your body, it also is correspondingly bound outside your skin. As far as your awareness can go into inner space, it can go that far outside your body. Since our chi and emotions can be blocked both internally and externally, it is possible to dissolve your chi and emotions inside and outside your physical body simultaneously.

Your emotional body extends into space much farther than your chi body. Adepts in both the East and West have developed techniques that enable people's minds to cover vast distances, so that individuals can be consciously aware of the wide-reaching effects of their emotional body far outside of their own physical space. The process of joining a human being with the Tao may be accomplished by connecting that which is inside a human being to the totality of the universe.

Your own emotional field is constantly mixing with other natural fields and other people's emotional fields at the level of energetic vibratory frequencies. You are constantly in contact with other fields, those of living entities and of natural phenomenon (such as mountains, oceans, and stars).* These fields have the capacity to activate your emotional energies without your knowing or even against your will unless mitigated, for example, by dissolving. When another energy field overlaps with your energy field, there are three basic possibilities: (1) that field will energize you positively; (2) it will bypass you like a gentle wind without any difficulty, as long as your energy is neutral and has no particular resonance with that field; or (3) if you have bound emotional energy inside or outside that resonates with the other field, it may interact with that blockage and negatively affect you through a chain reaction.

The chain reaction works like this: the incoming external energy activates your own bound negative emotional energy, reconfiguring your energy patterns and causing your energy channels to re-form in the pattern that you have during a negative emotional experience.** This change in

---

*The Chinese science *feng shui* is based on this premise. It seeks to mitigate the negative effects of environmentally occurring energy or to create positive energies not intrinsic to the locale.

**Actually, Taoists consider energy to be intrinsically neither positive nor negative. Energy does, however, configure our internal systems into reactions that are commonly held to be positive or negative, such as love, which makes us act and feel good, and frustration, which makes us feel and act badly.

your energetic configuration then activates your internal organs and glands to release all sorts of toxic substances inside your body, which in turn activate the brain to release more toxic substances. This process then sets the conditions for releasing and energizing destructive thought patterns. These thoughts further energize your channels and more deeply lock in your glands, internal organs, brain centers, and neural transmitters, and you find yourself in a negative chain reaction, with intensifying anger, frustration, greed, hate, and other so-called negative emotions. An opposite "positive" stimulation from sources outside you could also happen, inducing an energetic configuration stimulating hope, kindness, consideration, compassion, equanimity, forgiveness, and so on.

If you do not clear out your own energy fields beyond your body, then all energies coming in from an external environment can activate the unresolved energies in your own personal chi. In guitar playing, plucking one guitar string can induce a sympathetic vibration in another guitar string, with which it is not in physical contact. In like manner, an energetic frequency from outside your body can intensely activate a specific energy inside your body that would normally have remained inert or dormant. Your specific internal energy thus becomes active with respect to the specific events of your life occurring at the moment and makes a great deal of emotional noise. This reaction can cause you to be somewhat manipulated (as if you were a puppet) by the energy emanating from the huge chi fields of the stars.

The emotional energy you emanate also moves toward the stars and sooner or later returns back into your body, activating the emotional energies inside you, which are attached to your Consciousness. This activation causes or exacerbates mood swings or predispositions toward emotional states, both positive and negative. The energies of these moods are inside you, but without an external stimulus they might not have been awakened or strongly felt. They can remain hidden within the quiet desperation or confusion that sadly is all too often a fixture in the interior landscape of many people's minds. These astrologically induced energy flows can also affect the general physiology of a person for good or ill.

Astrology is based on such energetic interactions. The immensely strong energetic fields of the planets exert an ever-changing influence on the earth as they move through space. Such influence does not mean that events will necessarily occur, but it suggests that certain types of energy will be prevailing at a particular time, affecting the first six of your eight bodies.* Astrological influences can be overridden by clearing out blockages in your emotional body. Such clearing can be accomplished while sitting or while practicing tai chi chuan, ba gua, chi gung, or Taoist yoga. When you start clearing your emotional blockages it is important to tap directly into your glandular system, as well as into your internal organs. There are so many techniques available that the right one to be employed at any time depends on what is appropriate for a particular type of person or a certain situation. It is not really useful simply to talk about this or that technique in a cookbook approach. Human beings are too complicated to work that way.

Emotions and Emptiness

As you clear out the bound energy of your emotional body, you may find that emotions of anger dissolve and leave emotions of fear, which dissolve and leave emotions of insecurity, and so on. There is no predetermined sequence of emotions. Explore your own nature, remembering that it will take time and effort to resolve your personal problems. Once you are able to trace bound emotional energy back to its source, however, you will reach a point where you have access to the core of your being. At this point, you will begin to experience the early phases of what the Taoists call *emptiness*. Like flickering shadows from a candle, you will

*Individuality and the Tao are the two bodies not affected.

begin to get glimpses of and viscerally realize that there is something inside you that is beyond your personality, emotions, and the thoughts in your head.

At this depth, your emotional problems can suddenly become resolved, and you can reconnect these emotions to the core of your being. This reconnecting allows the energy of your emotions to be absorbed by your core, and from there to recirculate freely in your system. As long you have bound emotions, you are deprived of the positive potential of that energy, since it is separated from the core of your essence.

As you dissolve your bound emotional energy, your understanding of yourself will steadily increase. As you untie each emotional knot, it will seem as if it was never there in the first place. The Taoist water method of dissolving bound emotions is the exact opposite of the cathartic methods of other traditions, in which you express the emotions overtly and dramatically. The water Taoists prefer the dissolving method because it thoroughly removes all traces of the blocked emotions quietly and gently without drama, while promoting inner and outer peace and harmony with the world.

Taking Personal Responsibility for Doing Meditation

What does committing yourself to work on your emotional energy with meditation really mean? For thousands of years, the genuine mystic meditation traditions have had strict specifications for who should and should not be taught—whether or not a student was "worthy" or ready. In our modern mass market, consumer-oriented "democratic" societies, the concept of worthiness seems passé, especially when so many self-proclaimed gurus are selling enlightenment to whomever will buy.

In Taoism, the tradition of the student being "worthy" is especially critical in terms of the student's personal safety and wellbeing. It is also critical in terms of determining whether or not the student has a realistic chance of success in realizing the Tao in one lifetime. In the pre-electronic world, when people had more time to spend with each other, the process of learning how to take emotional responsibility for oneself was taught by the stable social institutions of the family and the church. These institutions are now rapidly breaking down. The coherent emotional education services and discipline these institutions once provided have been professionalized, taken over by the new priests of our age: the psychotherapists. Often, they are the only ones left to teach emotional responsibility.

If students are not capable of taking responsibility for their emotions, they are unprepared to evolve spiritually past a certain point.* Continuing to go deeper inside themselves and meditate will cause them to undergo needless mental and emotional tribulation. Students will think they just need to meditate more, when what they really need is external psychotherapy. If taking full responsibility for your emotions is not yet within your capacity, psychotherapy may be one of the only accessible places left where you can learn something about your emotions. You have to be careful because, in Taoist or any other powerful forms of meditation, when you really open up into the inner core of your mind and soul, a lack of emotional awareness can sometimes lead you into mental waters that are difficult to navigate.

In the Taoist meditative tradition, to qualify as a "worthy" student one had to take responsibility for the emotions arising within and not put them off on anything external. Students holding this value would then be able to use their emotional energy to resolve their inner conflicts responsibly without becoming self-destructive or blaming or attacking others for being the cause of their misery. In some Zen communities, for example, many students reach a stage of sitting practice where they are advised to seek out

---

*This is why, for example, in the stricter schools of the kabalistic tradition, which is the foundation of most of the Western mystic schools, members were not allowed into its deeper studies until after they were forty and had emotionally matured.

psychotherapy rather than continue meditating. This suggestion is made because, when one goes into powerful meditation states, such as emptiness or nonidentification with the body, emotions, or personality, incredible energies of the soul are released and, with them, one's suppressed emotional dysfunctions.

Traditionally, Taoist meditators know that these energies are personalized ghosts or demons and, with patience, forbearance, and gentleness, begin the process of applying the meditative effort to resolving the internal knots appearing in the consciousness. Some individuals, who come from extremely dysfunctional emotional backgrounds and who do not know how to take responsibility for their own emotions, either lash out at others or go partially mad or catatonic. For such severe needs, a psychotherapist is more appropriate than a meditation master. In the complex modern world, Taoist meditation is essentially for healthy, functional human beings who want to become completely clear. It is not for humans who are looking for a cheap form of psychological therapy. Presently in the West there are no Taoist communities, retreat centers, or monasteries that have the facilities or the economic support to give dysfunctional people the time, energy, and personal attention that the traditional monasteries in China could offer.

For individuals undergoing "a dark night of the soul," traditional meditation communities, ashrams, and monasteries historically provided a safe environment where the individual's food, clothing, and shelter were taken care of. There, individuals–with the full support of the community–could go through the madness and come out the other side to arrive at a level of permanently improved mental health or mystic awareness. Often, an individual or group of "caretaker" monks or adepts were on hand to monitor meditators. If meditators were unable to overcome their karmic obstacles and stayed mad, at least they were taken care of for life.

In the Western world, these support systems are currently virtually nonexistent. Many people in all the traditional Eastern and Western meditation schools experience, for varying lengths of time, this "dark night of the soul." In a meditation community I visited in India in the 1970s, for example, new members were encouraged or required to take part in psychotherapy groups to learn the capacity to take responsibility for their emotions before they were initiated as full-time members of the spiritual community. The psychological learning and therapy process provided people with a finer ability to (1) recognize boundaries; (2) feel their emotions and emotional nuances; (3) comprehend the devious nature of emotional suppressions; (4) become aware of the powerful effects unrecognized suppressed emotions can have on one's daily life; and (5) experience that emotional suppressions can realistically be gone through with the individual beneficially cleansed, liberated, and matured by the process.

The Taoists are known in China for their practical mysticism. They were convinced, by millennia of experience, that if you wish to go to the roots of your emotions (rather than just doing concentration exercises, repeating incantations, or engaging in functionless rituals) then you must bring a down-to-earth, long-term perspective to your practice. Rome was not built in a day. Freeing up the bound energetic tendencies toward needlessly convoluted emotions–tendencies that were created over lifetimes–can take a good deal of time.

How to Prevent Problems Arising from Meditation

Deep inside many human minds exist emotions and mental states that are disturbing. The process of meditation seeks to resolve those energies. Sometimes genuine spiritual meditation is like opening Pandora's box. When an individual encounters emptiness, repressed demons are released, which then come openly into our waking consciousness, resulting in powerful mood swings. Any latent mental or emotional problems you may have can begin to manifest–always a possibility for anyone engaging in any form of spiritual meditation.

The best situation is to have an exceptional teacher/adept guiding you in close, near-daily contact, along with support from an equally fine group of talented senior students–a rare configuration in today's world. Classically, the Taoists found there were some good precautions to prevent potential meditation problems from getting started in the first place, especially for those with a minimal external support system.

1. Never take yourself to the extremes of your concentration; 50-70 percent is fine. This 70 percent is a variable quantity, relative to your capacities at a given practice session. Tiredness and mental strain manifest well before you reach 100 percent of your mental stamina. On one day, the point before the mental strain appears (that is, when you exceed 70 percent) may be five to ten minutes. On other days, a half hour, or two or three hours. On some days, five hours. In all cases, the mind and brain must not be pushed to the point of strain, tension, or obsession. By adhering to this simple rule, the stamina of your concentration will most likely not exceed the capacity of your body/mind to absorb and process all the rising demons from your unconscious mind. On some days your concentration may take a quantum leap. If this is true, you still must not overstrain relative to your subjective experience of what internal strain is for you personally.

2. Accept that you are a human being with human capacities and don't feel you have to transform the whole of your life in one given day. It will take time. Try not to confuse obsession with tenacity. Obsession causes very real problems.

3. When finishing meditation, rub your hands vigorously and, beginning with your hands touching the crown of your head, bring your hands down all the areas of your head (front, back, and sides) and down to your chest or belly, so as to bring any chi

caught in the brain back down into the body. Energy caught in the brain after meditating tends to cause an overheating that can weaken nerves or cause disassociation.

4. Starting with sittings of only twenty minutes, do not increase your meditation time by more than five minutes a month. If you break a meditation routine for a long time, begin again at twenty minutes and work upward.

5. Avoid irregular marathon sessions (hours on end) unless under the personal supervision of a meditation master who can tell how much you can safely take. A sudden release of the deeply repressed material in the human mind, brought on by an excessive, unsupervised practice, is a common source of mental and emotional destabilization. If you have no stamina buildup from regular practice, your situation could become analogous to the "weekend warrior" athlete who damages his body by a short burst of sudden unprepared athletic training. Here, however, it is the mind, emotions, and central nervous system that are being pushed beyond their capacities.

By following these simple safety precautions, you can practice meditation confidently. If, however, at any time you have questions about your own emotional or mental states, err on the side of caution. Seek advice from a professional therapist who is sympathetic to the concept of meditation and who can give you a clear, honest reflection of the condition of your mind and emotions.

What Is Taoist Sexual Meditation?

CHAPTER
6

Lao Tse Tao Te Ching, Verse 2

*The gateways of the mysterious yin
Are the roots of Heaven and Earth*

What Is Taoist Sexual Meditation?

Since the dawn of time a continuum of beliefs has always existed concerning the meanings and permissible rules of sexual engagement. At one end of the continuum, sex is seen as a nasty business, bordering on evil, to be engaged in as little as possible, and then only according to the rules of the prevailing religion. At the other end of the continuum, consensual sex between a man and a woman is viewed as a healthy, normal human activity, a celebration of the life force. Sex has the potential to be either wonderful or a mess, depending on the sanity, internal balance, and openness of the participants.

Westerners often impute all sorts of meanings to normal consensual sex, but to the Taoists, sex is only another chi or meditation practice–it is not considered prurient or nonspiritual in any philosophical sense. The practice of Taoist meditation is basically the same regardless of modality; that is, you can meditate while standing, sitting, moving, lying down, or engaging in sexual activity. Sexual practices fit in neither the easier nor more difficult category, as during sex your body posture may be standing or sitting, moving or motionless. As a practice, sexual meditation is easier than sitting and moving meditations. However, the sexual methods are not as dependable as the standing and sitting practices, which the sexual methods support and accelerate. In the middle-level dissolving and advanced alchemical practices, it is hard to say where the balance lies. It depends on how naturally comfortable and relaxed you are with sex.

During sexual activity most people become more fully alive, the energy of the body becomes flush, and the mind and emotions soar. For many people, it is easier to feel and influence the body's energies and physical tissues during sexual play than at any other time. Sex can unleash the procreative force, which also unleashes human creativity and awareness. However, a certain percentage of the population will always find it more comfortable to access the chi within through solo meditative means rather than through the duality of sexual meditation.

Through passionate sex, your innate physical and psychic capacities start to become accessible naturally. Consequently, for many people the sexual act naturally enhances their awareness of chi sensations to which they were numb before. If you keep your awareness open while making love, you can begin to feel the different kinds of physical and energetic blockages inside your system. You can then learn to direct your own internal energy generated from lovemaking into an injured or diseased part of your body, to dissolve and heal. In like manner, you can also direct your partner's sexual energy to "loop into" your blockages to aid in dissolving them. Conversely, your partner can direct his or her energy toward helping your particular problem. You can then mutually dissolve any blocked energy that happens to exist in either of your bodies.

The core of sexual meditation involves adapting the Taoist meditative dissolving practice to lovemaking. Once you have linked your consciousness to that of your sexual partner, your mind can go into his or her mindstream for the purpose of dissolving any blockages in the entwined energetic system the two of you have become. The smoothest way on the face of the earth to achieve direct contact with the consciousness of another is through making love. Taoists believe it takes much more skill, psychic power, and finesse to gain such contact with another person when separate than through meditative sex. The reason is that, in sexual involvement, energy is increased and immediate—everything is "right there."

FOCUS ON A SPECIAL TOPIC
How This Material Was Learned

 I originally heard about Taoist sexual meditation in the late 1960s from one of my first internal arts teachers in Taiwan. He introduced me to a secret Taoist sex cult whose practices would have made the wildest of hippies blush, even during the height of that generation's sexual revolution.

After hearing from one of his other students who worked in my thin-walled hotel that I obviously enjoyed sex, the master said to me during one of our private classes, "So you are a young man who is enthusiastic about sex. But do you know really how to do it?" Indignant, I replied, "I beg your pardon. What the hell are you talking about?" Over the next few years, he made it pretty clear that, except for a lot of youthful enthusiasm that doesn't last all that long, I did not have the faintest clue about sex.

The master explained that whereas animals merely join genitals during sex, human beings have the ability to add other pleasurable enjoyment to the sexual act. To start, he taught me how to develop hand sensitivity, which is extremely important not only for sexuality but for tai chi and Chinese therapeutic bodywork as well. Both male and female genitals require handling with sensitivity and adroitness, whether such touching occurs during mutual sex play or solo masturbation. The means for achieving this sensitivity are set forth in this chapter, along with other Taoist physical, energetic, and dissolving exercises. Many of these techniques may be practiced solo; a few require partners.

Energetic Intimacy Is Not Based on Length of Relationship

Many people find it both uncomfortable and difficult to open up sexually and emotionally to someone of the opposite sex. The religious and romantic traditions of the West allow individuals to feel more loving only toward a "special other" they have actually married, romantically bonded with, or have known for a long time. But the Taoists believe you can have a sexual encounter with someone you met just fifteen minutes ago, and if you have the ability to fully open your spirit during lovemaking, you can experience incredible nonattached, unconditional emotional love toward that "stranger."

The capacity of your heart and your being to open to another has nothing to do with how long the two of you have shared time together, be it one second or one hundred years. It has everything to do with the degree to which you are willing to let your essence open to the other. It is possible for two people who have known each other for only an hour before going to bed to have more genuine intimacy than a couple who have been together for fifty years.

In one sense, what happens during lovemaking is timeless. From the standpoint of sexual meditation, it is necessary that practitioners be emotionally, mentally, and psychically naked in front of each other. Your physical body is only a surface part of you; emotions can affect you much more strongly than your physical body. The question is, Can you release the actual emotions you have inside yourself–meaning, can you fully share your emotions, mind, and psyche with your lover? The next question then becomes, Are you willing to feel what the other–your lover–is going through? If you can answer yes to these questions (that is, you are willing to fulfill these two conditions), then you and your partner can help dissolve each other's internal blockages, making your sexual encounter a mutually absorbing and freeing experience.

Why the Taoist Practices Must Be Successively Learned One by One

In all forms of Taoist meditation, physical and chi practices, such as chi gung, are necessary preparation for learning emotional energy practices. Work with the emotions, in turn, precedes work with the other five of your eight bodies, where the quality of energy becomes significantly more refined. The same sequence applies to sexual meditation practices as well. Taking into account the whole range of human energies, emotional energy is a relatively gross phenomenon. It is critical that a person become stable, open, balanced, and mature in the energy of his or her body, chi, and emotions before embarking on work in the higher levels. It can take as much as five to ten years to become stable at the level of body and chi, which is why in the classical tradition chi gung was practiced before Taoist meditation, and why sexual chi gung was learned before sexual meditation.

Once you have done your preparatory chi practices, however, it is critical to open up fully and clear your overt and subliminal emotions. Why? So you can experientially feel and develop some emotional intelligence, rather than merely possess a disassociated mental construct of emotion, before going on to the psychic stage of practice. If this is not accomplished, real problems can crop up downstream. A great difficulty that many have, especially men, is that instead of experiencing emotions directly, they *think about what they feel emotionally*. When you begin to access the emotional body, thinking about rather than feeling emotions leads to an inability to know what is happening inside you. This failure to experience emotions directly causes an individual's deeper emotional garbage to spew out unconsciously, rather than consciously, a process that can turn people into unfeeling monsters.

Without the capacity to feel emotion, it is nearly impossible to have true humility. Without the presence of genuine emotional grounding from the psychic level, we are capable of looking at human beings as mere "ants," as did the gods of ancient Greece, who played with mortals in cruel and capricious ways. The ego at the psychic level is extremely subtle, without many of the landmarks of normal behavior that give perspective to life. For that reason, the ability to distinguish between your emotional and mental bodies is a necessary attainment that you must gain before entering the psychic world.

This statement is especially true for the sexual practices, in which you can progress internally at accelerated speed. As in the other forms of Taoist meditation, you must first be reasonably mature emotionally before embarking on the practices for the higher bodies.

Sexual Chi Gung

Chi gung practitioners have been doing a certain tendon-loosening and hand-strengthening physical exercise since time immemorial. This exercise makes the hands, fingers, tendons, and joints very strong, loose, and flexible. Besides helping to prevent and mitigate hand arthritis, assuring fast-moving fingers and a strong grip, and improving finger skills for musicians, this exercise will give each of your fingers the sensitivity, speed, stamina, and reflexes needed for prolonged effective manual stimulation of your lover during foreplay. For many people, after only five minutes of manual stimulation, the tendons of the hand shorten, causing cramps (sometimes quite painful) in the palm and fingers. Such cramping causes progressive loss of ability to move the fingers with sensitivity. One undesirable result of this is that some people may not engage in foreplay to the extent necessary to "warm up" their partner's body from an energetic standpoint.

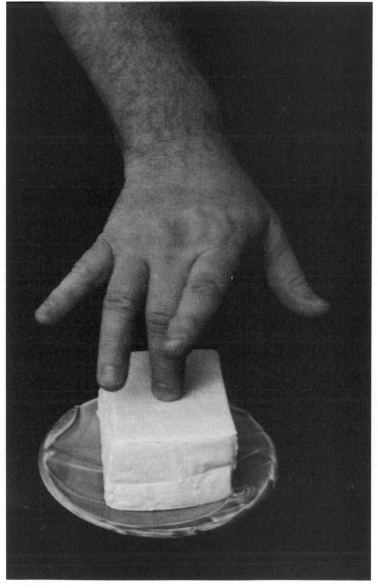

Photo courtesy of Michael McKee

Using tofu to develop hand sensitivity (see page 165).

FOCUS ON PRACTICE
Finger Rolling

This exercise is done alone in two phases. Phase 1 has three parts. Do each hand in turn.

Phase 1
Part 1: Fingers Move to the Thumb **(Fig. 9)**

1. Hold your thumb fixed in space above the middle of your palm.

2. Starting with your little finger and progressing to your index finger **(Figs. 9a–d)**, move each fingertip in a rolling motion so that each touches your steady thumb tip in turn. Do this five times. Concentrate on rolling your fingers slowly and rhythmically.

3. Next, repeat the same action in the opposite direction, starting from your index finger and finishing with your little finger.

4. Progress to having your fingertips touch your thumb more quickly and fluidly, as you stretch the insides of your hands upward from the base of the palms to the fingertips.

FOCUS ON PRACTICE
Finger Rolling (continued)

Figure 9 Finger Rolling Exercise

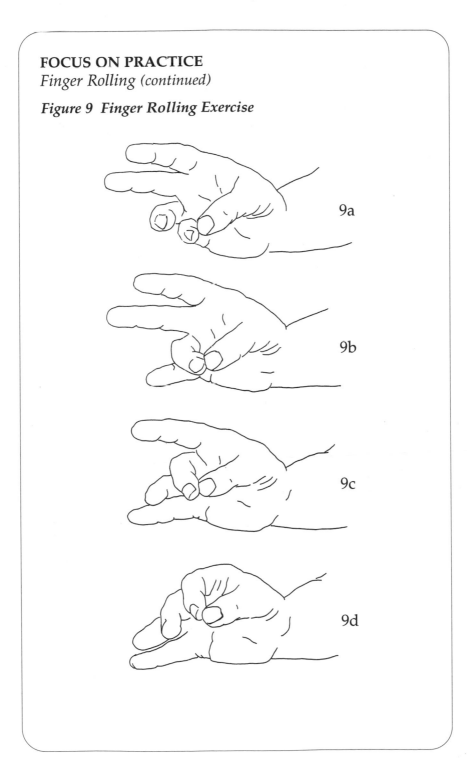

9a

9b

9c

9d

FOCUS ON PRACTICE
Finger Rolling (continued)

Part 2: Thumb Moves to the Fingers
1. Curve your palm so the little finger is well within the borders of your palm and not toward or beyond the fleshy edge of your palm.
2. Move your thumb so that its tip touches the other four fingertips, one by one, beginning with the little finger and moving toward the index finger **(Figs. 10a–d)**. The fingertips are held still. First move your thumb slowly and then more quickly and fluidly, stretching your muscles and tendons all the way from your wrist to your fingertips.
3. After your thumb touches your index finger, let it continue as far to the side as possible, stretching the whole hand before circling back to again touch your little finger **(Fig. 10e)**.

After a significant number of repetitions, repeat the exercise in the reverse direction. Touch your index fingers first, little finger last, and as before continue to move your thumb and spread your hand open.

Part 3: Combining the Two Moves
After you have separately mastered the finger and thumb motions of parts 1 and 2, combine these together into one continuous movement, as follows. Begin by touching your little finger first and index finger last. After five times, repeat the same process, only reverse directions and begin touching your index finger first and little finger last.
1. Fingers move: Begin with your little finger and touch each of your four fingertips one by one to your thumb (held fixed in space above your palm). After your index finger has touched your thumb, stretch open your hand wide. Again sequentially touch your four fingers to your thumb, and again stretch your hand to the maximum, and repeat.
2. Thumb moves: Then without stopping or resting your hand, if possible, continue in the other direction as your thumb touches your index finger first and your little finger last, doing all the motions of part 2.

FOCUS ON PRACTICE
Finger Rolling (continued)

Figure 10 Thumb Rolling Exercise

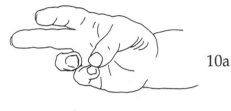

10a

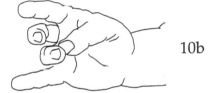

10b

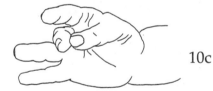

10c

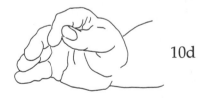

10d

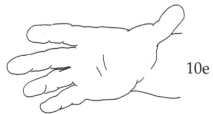

10e

Do ten repetitions initially (five in one direction, five in the other). Then work your way up to one hundred or more over time. This exercise develops tremendous finger dexterity. It also beneficially stimulates and builds up the chi of your internal organs, as the acupuncture meridians of all your internal organs end in the fingertips.

Phase 2
1. Repeat phase 1, part 1, but instead of touching the tip of your thumb, the fingertips now touch the base of the thumb or at least the big muscle below your thumb.
2. Repeat phase 1, part 2, but now the thumb tip touches the base of your fingers, rather than their tips. The number of repetitions remains the same.

The stretch of your hand muscles, ligaments, and tendons should not only include your palm but also extend all the way down to your forearm.

The Importance of Hand and Finger Sensitivity in Sexual Play

The manual stimulation of male and female genitals requires a great deal of sensitivity. Insensitive or gross tactile behavior during sex usually inhibits the full potential of the sexual response. With greater hand sensitivity, you can feel accurately what your partner is going through and can adjust to his or her changing sexual responses. A sensitive touch enables both women and men to discriminate between insufficient finger pressure and overstimulation. Developing this sensitivity can be essential, because people of both sexes frequently do not externally reveal discomforts they may experience during lovemaking.

Hand sensitivity brings deeper levels of sensuality. Many women enjoy playing with the different kinds of hardness and skin texture changes that occur in the penis during fondling; many men enjoy playing with the different textures of the vagina. The genitalia of both sexes have zones that tap directly into the energies of the mind, body, and spirit. Knowledge of these zones can greatly enhance sexual pleasure. When caressing sexual organs, it is a good idea to be sensitive to the surrounding pubic area. Is it becoming overly tense? Is your partner's body developing a resistance to your touch? If so, this can diminish the sexual experience and possibly lead to emotional difficulties between the two of you after the sex is over.

How does either partner know when to increase, decrease, or keep the same level of stimulation? Instructing each other during lovemaking is one way, but often in full sexual flush the pleasurable body sensations get so strong that talk can negatively alter the excitability of the mind and the genital nerves–the mood may break. It is far better to train your nonverbal sense of touch to let it tell you what is going on. The hand sensitivity and manual stimulation techniques presented in this chapter offer such training.

FOCUS ON PRACTICE
Using Tofu to Develop Hand Sensitivity

 One of the best supplementary trainings for developing sexual hand sensitivity involves tofu, whose texture and density (both hard and soft varieties) closely approximates that of human flesh.

There are essentially only three ways to apply effective motion or pressure on the penis, clitoris, and vaginal walls: (1) on a line either up and down or back and forth (that is, side to side); (2) with circular and figure-eight movements; and (3) tapping (applying pressure and quickly releasing) in either rhythmic or arrhythmic ways–which is usually not as effective as methods 1 and 2, unless your hands are incredibly sensitive. All three methods can be practiced on tofu.

Begin your finger sensitivity training by first using your middle or index finger. Eventually, progress until you are able to use any or all of the fingers of your hand, including your thumbs. Keep contact on the same patch of tofu surface without

FOCUS ON PRACTICE
Using Tofu to Develop Hand Sensitivity (continued)

sliding off until you have finished the exercise. Repeat the exercise by moving your finger to a new patch of tofu surface.

1. Touch the top surface of a smooth cake of tofu with either your middle or your index finger as lightly as possible. Adjust your finger pressure and adhesion so you can grip the skin of the tofu without sliding or breaking the bean curd's skin.
2. Vary your hand pressure to penetrate the "flesh" and cause the tofu to move, layer by layer, deeper toward the bottom, until you can make the whole cake move with a very light touch on the same patch of skin on the surface.
3. In the beginning, you will probably be able to get the whole tofu cake to move only as a single unit. With time and copious practice, however, you will be able to identify exactly which layer of the tofu your finger pressure will move. Stay with it until you can move one specific layer only, leaving the rest of the cake unaffected.
4. Apply what you have learned on the tofu to various erogenous zones of your partner, including the genitals. You will find that the nerve sensitivity you are acquiring will, with practice, easily transfer to your mouth and tongue. When you learn to feel in one place, it makes it easier to feel in another.

In the back-and-forth flux of lovemaking, it may be either a lighter or heavier pressure that will stimulate the nerves of the genitals more deeply or more toward the surface. The ability to touch the surface of the skin and be able to project your physical chi and consciousness awareness via your touch to various layers beneath is a basic sexual chi gung skill (as well as a primary skill in the healing massage work called chi gung tui na). If you practice regularly with tofu, within a year you should be able to use your fingers to stimulate erogenous zones for a prolonged time without strain.

The Nature of Yin and Yang Energy

Classic Taoist philosophy states that men and women have energetic sexual differences. The Taoists believe that after a woman fully activates her female yin energy and a man fully activates his male yang energy, then and only then is it possible for men and women to completely appreciate and embody their opposite energy within themselves. So in Taoist thought, the primary functions of yin and yang energy differ. Yang energy characteristically tends to go in an outward direction, like fire or a beam of light. The opposite is true for yin energy, which characteristically tends to flow inward, to absorb, like earth and water; yin energy wants to allow something to come into it, to let that something manifest and emerge, become nourished, and grow. Whereas the creative outflowing yang energy does not mind destruction, the inflowing yin energy loves growth and loathes destruction.

Taoist thought holds that a woman's heart center, or middle tantien, is naturally more alive and activated than a man's; correspondingly, a man's lower tantien is naturally more activated than a woman's. The heart center is ruler of human emotions; the lower tantien governs physicality.

A woman's sexual energy concentrates in the lower, yin part of her body–that is, her feet, ankles, knees, thighs, and buttocks. Regardless of which sexual foreplay or dissolving technique is used, the lower portion of her body is where the man must physically and energetically turn her on and keep her turned on before and during sexual intercourse. The more intensely the energy accumulates in a woman's feet, the stronger her orgasms can be. A woman wants her yin sexual energy to move from being centered in her vagina down to her feet. In the beginning of foreplay, the man should play with the woman's feet, kissing and sucking her toes, in order to draw her sexual energy down to her feet and below her feet to the end of her etheric body. Once her yin energy is warmed up, it can be moved upward to anywhere in the upper yang part of her body.

A man is the opposite. Regardless of which sexual foreplay or dissolving technique is used, for a woman to excite a man and maintain his erection, she should concentrate his sexual energy in the upper, yang part of his body (that is, his kidneys, upper torso, arms, and head) before playing with his genitals, buttocks, and legs. For a man's sexual energy to reach its strongest levels of intensity, he wants it to transfer from his genitals and rise to his upper back and the crown of his head and above his head, to the endpoint of his etheric body. In the beginning of foreplay, the woman should first kiss or suck the man's fingers, arms, neck, ears, nose, forehead, or top of his head. Once he is turned on, she can move down to his lower body.

Chi Gung Energetic Anatomy of the Male Genitals

Along the penis, from the base of its shaft to the tip of its head, are zones that correspond energetically to different internal organs, energy channels, and energy centers in the body, as the accompanying chart illustrates.

Relationship of Zones of the Penis to a Man's Body

This zone of the penis will activate	this energetic aspect
the base of the shaft	the lower tantien
the middle of the shaft	the middle tantien
the entire head of the penis	the upper tantien
the skin around the penis or glans (if present)	the physical body
the center of the shaft	the central energy channel
slightly in from the surface toward the center of the shaft	the etheric body
slightly deeper in from the surface toward the center of the shaft	the emotional body
the left side of the shaft	the left energy channel
the right side of the shaft	the right energy channel
the entire head of the penis	all the yang meridians
the base of the shaft	all the yin meridians

Relationship of Zones of the Vagina to a Woman's Body

This zone of the vagina will activate	this energetic aspect
the opening of the cervix	the central channel
the vaginal canal (where the cervix sits)	the upper tantien
the middle of the vaginal canal	the middle tantien
the entrance to the vaginal canal	the lower tantien
the left side of the vagina	the left channel
the right side of the vagina	the right channel
the top (end) of vaginal canal	the body of the Tao
ring 1	the body of individuality
ring 2	the causal body
ring 3	the psychic body
ring 4	the mental body
ring 5	the emotional body
ring 6	the chi body
ring 7	the physical body

Chi Gung Energetic Anatomy of the Female Genitals

Along its length, the vagina possesses zones that energetically correspond to and activate different internal organs, energy channels, and energy centers in the body, as the accompanying chart illustrates. The "rings" are progressive regions that extend around the entire circumference of the vagina, like stacked coins, from the cervix to the vulva.

If you wish to waken, rather than deaden, the more subtle energies of your sexual partner, it is necessary to pay attention to activating all the various energetic sections of the genital area during foreplay and intercourse.

FOCUS ON PRACTICE
Transferring Sexual Energy around Your Body

 This solo sexual chi gung exercise replicates energy movements you can use when engaged in intercourse. Place your hands lightly on your genitals. Women should not physically penetrate the vagina but should use only enough pressure to feel the energy of the hand going into the vagina. Using your mind, take the energy from your hand and do this exercise in three progressive stages.

1. With your mind, dissolve your hand.
2. Without force, start opening and closing your inguinal region, or kwa, as you pull energy in and out of your hand. When transferring energy around your body you may choose to use one of two possible pathways: the micro-cosmic orbit (up the spine and down the front center line of the body) or the central channel (see Appendix D for location of the kwa and energy channels).
   - Or pull your dissolved energy from your hands into your genitals then into and up your spine (that is, from your genitals to your perineum, to your tailbone, and up your spine).
   - Or pull your chi from your genitals to your perineum, up your central energy channel, and into your lower tantien.

FOCUS ON PRACTICE
Transferring Sexual Energy around Your Body (continued)

- Push the chi from your spine or lower tantien to your genitals and with your hand pull the energy back into your hand.
- Move your dissolved energy rhythmically back and forth between your genitals and your spine or lower tantien until it flows smoothly, with minimal effort.

3. Use the tip of the penis or opening to the vagina to pull the energy from your hand into your genitals and up the central channel to the tantien and crown of the head. Or move the energy from the perinium and tailbone through the ming men on the spine, and up the spine to the crown of the head. Then continue to pull energy down either your central channel (if you are more advanced) or down the conception vessel on your body's front center line, down to your lower tantien, and return it back to your genitals and into your hand.

4. Push your lower tantien's chi out from your genitals into your hands, and project that energy up your arm. Move it from the wrist to the elbow, to the shoulder, to the spine and neck, to the top of your head, down either the central channel or the spine to the tailbone, down to the perineum and continuing up to your genitals, where you complete the circuit in your hand.

It is very important that you move your energy gently, without force. Forcing your energy or your mind during sex results in nerves getting exhausted sooner rather than later. When sex becomes a forced exercise, it becomes more of a power trip, much different from something sensual, erotic, or meditative.

Taoist Sexual Meditation Techniques

CHAPTER 7

Lao Tse Tao Te Ching, Verse 7

Why can Heaven and Earth last long and endure?
It is because they do not live for themselves alone

Taoist Sexual Meditation Techniques

Shifting the Yang Fire of the Eyes

From the Taoist perspective, for most women the emotional content of sex is more important than the physical. For this reason, Taoists believe, many women in the aftermath of a sexual encounter will bond emotionally more easily than will men, who often will simply be satisfied from the physical act alone. For most men, it takes time to get past the physical and into the deeper, emotional side of sex. The priorities of yang and yin energy, as manifested in male and female humans, are different.

Most men respond sexually to the energy they feel in their eyes. A man sees an attractive woman and immediately responds. If a woman wants to activate the emotional side of a man's sexual response, as opposed to the physical side, she should activate his heart center fully and then raise that heart energy right up to his eyeballs. A direct channel of energy links the heart center to the eyes and upper tantien; if a woman can help a man activate that channel and thereby reduce his "yang fire of the eyes," she can significantly increase his emotional lovemaking response.

This method can normally enhance the emotional experience, either immediately or over time. Suppose energetic foreplay does not culminate in intercourse and the man falls asleep. If the woman has activated the man's channel from his heart to his eyes, the man will be more predisposed to sharing sexual emotional energy when he wakes up, or at least gradually more and more, day by day, in a long-term relationship.

Using this technique, a woman will feel two kinds of flutter in a man's heart. The first will have a quality of holding something in, a spasm-like quality. Keep playing with this flutter until it softens and releases. The second flutter will be as if something wants to flow but can't quite. For this flutter, give your lover some encouragement and keep on moving the energy of the flutter along until it goes to his eyes. How? Be creative, in every way you can! You could for example focus on either his physical or etheric body by using your mind intent, sound, or body parts ranging from your eyes, hands and tongue, to your erogenous zones to allow this to occur. However, if a man does not like having his energy moved between his heart and eyes, he can easily find a way to stop you.

Physical Foreplay

Important Points for Men

For many women, penetration of the penis into the vagina alone will not awaken a capacity for orgasm. A substantial number of women cannot achieve orgasm without manual or oral stimulation. Caring and gentleness, along with sensitive finger, mouth, and tongue technique, can be extremely helpful for such women. Once the nervous system relaxes sufficiently, however, and the woman's body is capable of achieving orgasm through manual or oral stimulation, she will usually be able to experience orgasms during intercourse. Men frequently do not realize that if the pelvic nerves do not relax and release at a deep level, a woman will remain nonorgasmic; tension defeats relaxation.

The main vaginal stimulation point that ultimately causes a woman to have an orgasm may be called the "spot."

The "spot" could be the clitoris, G-spot, or anywhere in the vagina that brings the woman to orgasm. The "spot" is not fixed–it continuously shifts anywhere within an area the size of an American quarter. A woman may be progressively turned on by a man's fingers on the spot. If fingers linger there too long, however, the situation of "too much of a good thing" might apply, causing the woman's nerves to become overstimulated and numb. Sexual frustration caused by "being so close and yet so far away" is unsatisfying for both parties involved.

It is helpful to understand the mechanism of a woman's vaginal/clitoral (spot) stimulation pattern. When manually stimulating any place in a woman's vagina, especially the clitoris, think of the exact orgasm-bringing stimulation point–the "spot"–as the epicenter of an earthquake. If a stone is thrown into a still pond of water, rings spread out from the epicenter. In like manner, a series of energetic rings extends from the orgasmic epicenter of the vagina to the edge of the outermost ring. These rings have a variable depth of about an inch and circumference approximating that of an American quarter. Within this circumference are five to ten concentric rings that can be clearly differentiated by sensitive fingers and tongue.

Through practice (along with the sensitivity gained through the tofu training technique in the previous chapter), a man can achieve the skill of isolating each ring independently. The "spot" may shift, and a man may need to follow it to its new ring location. Do not continue to stimulate a "spot" that has moved on; that stimulation is now creating numbness or pain instead of pleasure. A variety of tactile combinations will bring your partner closer to or farther away from orgasm. The range includes going faster with lighter or heavier finger pressure, slower with deeper or lighter pressure, staying still and just gently vibrating your finger, staying on one "spot," or moving between different rings and "spots." Adjust your touch sensitively according to her needs. In general, the clitoris and "spot" are more sensitive to stimulation than the walls of the vagina; nonetheless, the vagina and cervix are exceptionally orgasmic in some women.

If the woman is tense and you overstimulate one spot, her nerves there will deaden. She needs to relax. You should shift your fingers two or three rings distant from the over-stimulated spot to an understimulated area. This action may produce a new spot and an orgasm. If not, continue to stimulate this new area until you intuitively feel that the original spot has rested and can reawaken to pleasurable sexual sensation. Return to the original spot and start again. This could bring orgasm. If not, go back and forth between that which can be stimulated and that which needs rest, until your partner's nerves relax completely and she climaxes.

Rings of stimulation also exist externally, around the whole pubic mons area. These emanate from, and can bring energy into, the vagina, setting up a pre-orgasmic environment for genital stimulation. Sometimes, playing with this area alone can bring a woman to orgasm.

If the woman is already orgasmic, feel when her orgasm has completely released, and then allow her necessary rest and nerve regeneration before moving into another orgasm scenario. The time required for rest varies considerably from woman to woman and also changes during different stages of life.

Finally, it is good to remember that, if you want sex to proceed for a long time, you must become involved with the interplay of energy between you and your partner, rather than just focus on the desire to culminate the act with an orgasm.

Important Points for Women

Most women are unaware that a man can have a strong orgasm without ejaculating or a weak, nonpleasurable orgasm while emitting semen, or can have an erect penis that is numb to sensation or in a strained, painful state incapable of ejaculation. The male organ operates over a range of sensitivity. Like a woman's genitals, the penis needs to go through cycles of becoming excited and resting. If it cannot do this, its overstimulated nerves lock, ceasing to give pleasure and instead delivering pain, discomfort, and numbness, causing the penis to go flaccid. In fondling a man's genitals, a woman needs to consider certain factors. These include what kind of pressures cause the penis to get excited, whether the excitement generated will lead to a continuous pleasurable wave without ejaculation or to a rapid ejaculation, what rhythmic hand movements should be used, when it is better to stroke the base, middle, or head of the penis, and when the man requires a temporary rest.

FOCUS ON PRACTICE
Tongue Strengthening for Kissing and Oral Sex

When you use your tongue in sexual activity, one problem is that the area underneath the root of the tongue tends to fatigue, causing a negative cascade effect whereby the whole tongue and jaw muscles weaken, cramp, and lose sensitivity. Two useful solo exercises to remedy this problem follow. In doing these exercises, stretch your tongue as far outside your teeth as possible.

1. Move your tongue around in circles of varying size. Do this up and down, side to side, and diagonally at varying speeds for five to ten minutes. Such movement will start stretching the ligaments and will strengthen the muscles at the root of the tongue and jaw, enabling you to engage in oral sex for extended duration.

2. Curl the tongue outside the teeth. Alternate between the tip of your tongue touching your top and bottom lips and the sides of your mouth. Keep this tongue motion going in both directions for two to three minutes.

Tongue sensitivity, speed, and control are equally important for kissing and oral sex. To gain these attributes, you can practice the tofu sensitivity training in the previous chapter, substituting your tongue for your finger.

If a woman practices the tofu sensitivity training regularly, she should be able to stimulate a man's penis pleasurably for a prolonged time without either partner feeling strain. It is important to have a touching technique that does not restrict the small blood vessels in the testicles or penis.

The Problem of Sex, Nerves, and Stress: Taoist Remedies

In many preindustrial societies, a tired farmer or physical laborer who put in a twelve-hour day could still engage in sex all night. Although the bodies of these workers were tired, their nerves were not. Nerve fatigue causes lack of interest in sex and a lessening of ability to have sex.

In modern times, nervous exhaustion dulls or eliminates the sex drive by rendering the central nervous system in general and the sexual nerves in particular incapable of feeling and responding. Computers are a good example of the type of contemporary activity that can bring nervous rather than physical exhaustion. After continuous hours of excessive visual and mental overstimulation, anyone's nerves can become temporarily burnt out from the effects of a mind racing faster than the nervous system can handle. To help resolve this currently widespread problem we must turn our attention to relaxing, strengthening, and unjangling our nerves and opening our energy channels. The Taoist-based techniques in the "Focus on Practice" section opposite are a start in the right direction.

Partner Dissolving Exercises

These meditative partner dissolving exercises can be practiced in a sexual or nonsexual manner.* If no active sexual charge is present, however, the effect will be weaker than if the exercises are done sexually.

*They are commonly done nonsexually in chi gung tui na–Chinese energetic therapeutic massage.

FOCUS ON PRACTICE
Meditative Partner Techniques to
Reawaken Tired Sexual Nerves

One way of rejuvenating is for you and your partner to breath together, loudly enough so you can both hear each other. Continue until, gradually, your breaths synchronize. Slowly allow each breath to become deeper and quieter, until both of you grow very quiet inside and breathe as one person.

Another way for partners whose nerves are exhausted to bring each other to life is to hold and gently squeeze each other's hands, first lightly and then with more intensity as your sexual contractions begin to awake, until you both are pulsing together in unison. Keep the pulsing synchronized until your minds and nervous systems slow down and relax.

You can also simultaneously breathe and pulse hands in synchronization. Eventually, you will both become quiet, calm, and aware of the excitement and pleasure you are generating in each other's bodies. Let the nervous exhaustion fade away as you both relax into, and feel the interplay of, each other's yin and yang energy.

Pulsing is the body's basic condition during lovemaking. Pulsation occurs naturally in your genitals during pleasurable writhing and sexual contractions. The basic question is, Can you relax your nerves sufficiently so that you and your partner can pulse together? Commonly what happens to a lover who is exhausted is that he or she simply closes down, becomes numb, and verbally or nonverbally says "no, thank you" to sex. If both of you can breathe and pulse in unison, along with developing mutual sexual rapport, something else equally valuable can occur.

The process is similar to what occurs if you put your hand on a shaking, frightened animal and gently breathe and pulse with it. After a while the shaking will often stop.

Allow your partner the time to release nervous exhaustion. If after a few minutes of pulsing, and after some releases of accumulated nervous system tension, your partner is in the mood, enjoy. If he or she really wants to go to sleep or crawl into a cocoon, however, allow it. If in fifteen to twenty minutes awakening occurs from the deep state of relaxation your pulsing has induced, the odds are that sexual interest will be present.

Hand Holding

This exercise starts with the hands, which are easy to feel, and eventually extends to every body part.

1.   Hold hands. Both hands or only one hand may be used.
2.   Each of you should completely dissolve any blockages in your own hands, releasing any blocked energy you find there. (Inner or outer dissolving may be used.)
3.   After you have dissolved your own hand, dissolve the energy of your partner's hand.
4.   Now, each of you dissolve your own and the other's hand simultaneously.

One common side effect of this dissolving process is that you may start feeling your blood pumping more strongly. But also notice what are you feeling, what is happening inside yourself. Can you feel the sensations of your physical tissue only, or also the more subtle sensations of your chi, your emotions, or combinations thereof? Feel for the subtle sensations that are the precursors of full-body emotional experience. Trust yourself. If you're doubtful, don't worry about it. Right now, let this be a relaxed situation.

Let your mind and whole body relax as much as you can as you energetically sink into (that is, feel below the skin surface of) the other person's hand. Gradually let your mind go into something deeper than just the physical body. See if you can feel the bio-energy of your partner and, afterward, the emotions. Take a rest whenever you need to. Make this an adventure rather than a chore.

Foot Holding

This procedure is described from the point of view of the man holding the woman's foot (thereby activating her yin energy). Certainly, the reverse could be described, and many permutations and combinations are possible. For simplicity let's focus on one hand holding one foot.

1. The man and woman each respectively dissolve any blockages in their own hand and foot.
2. The man then dissolves his hand and the woman's foot; she dissolves her foot and his hand, both people gaining a sense of hand and foot merging.

The partners here must be capable of dissolving their hands and feet before moving on to dissolving the entire arm or leg of the other. This dissolving of a partner is the next more subtle level of the dissolving process. Your consciousness and awareness must now focus through your own body part into another's energy field.

Head Holding

Here we shift the focus to the woman holding the man's head and activating his yang energy.

1. The man dissolves the energy in his head.
2. The woman dissolves the energy in her own hand.
3. The woman dissolves her hand and the man's head, and the man dissolves his head and the woman's hand, with both people gaining a sense of hand and head merging.

If the man has a headache, he might find it partially or fully cured.

Energetic Boundaries Disappear

Focusing on the feet and head is merely the beginning of the partner dissolving exercises. An old phrase in Taoism says, "In the weaving back and forth between foreplay and intercourse, if you haven't touched every part of your lover's body, then you have not completed the experience." Making love is more than just genital rubbing. At some point in the process of lovemaking you want to have deliberately touched every single section of your partner's body. Allowing your mind to go into your partner's body/mind and vice versa causes your boundaries to disappear in a sea of energy. Consequently, you gain a whole new dimension to your intimate experience of your lover.

Spiritual Practice Is Different from Entertainment

Although pleasure is an essential part of the package, the genuine Taoist or tantric meditation traditions are based not on spiritual entertainment but on developing a personal relationship with Consciousness itself. Sex is a vehicle, as are standing, moving, sitting, and lying down, rather than an end in itself. There is no need to justify natural sexual urges under the guise of "spirituality." The Taoist position is that, if you only want to expand your horizons and have a more enriching, orgasmic good time with sex, learn sexual chi gung rather than sexual meditation.

The aim of sexual meditation is to have sex in a human fashion, with genuine sincerity and practice, ascending first to a stage of involvement with each other at least slightly above that of animals, and ultimately quite a bit further. Taoist morality dictates that you do not use sex to manipulate or harm others at any level. Keep in mind this variation on the Golden Rule: "Whatever you do to someone, you have just done to your Consciousness."

The long-range goal of Taoist sexual meditation is one thing: to take the raw material of physical sex and use it to actualize a person's potentialities of spirit and Consciousness.

The Complete Package Includes Both the Wonderful and the Frightening

When you do any Taoist practice, especially the sexual or other meditation work, the unexpected, both wonderful and frightening, is part of the package. Predictability has its time and place, but during sex you definitely want the unpredictable to keep surfacing, no matter what it is. If you get caught off guard, your body flutters, muscles twitch, or you feel weird physical sensations–fair enough, enjoy it. Sometimes, especially when psychic energy releases from the body, these sensations seem larger than life.

Understand that this is all just energy. We tend to place incredible value on what we think things mean. When you can learn instead to view the specific content of any kind of experience as merely an energy being expressed, your attachment to implications and potential meanings will diminish. Most experiences will cease to have overwhelming and perhaps destabilizing influence on you.

The one thing that must be realized is that when sex is used as an exceptionally intense meditation practice, you are forced to confront what is inside you. It may be fun or it may become problematic. It is largely up to you.

Advanced Taoist Sexual Meditation

Advanced Taoist sexual work primarily focuses on sexuality to fully awaken the spirit and Consciousness within. It involves complex esoteric sexual meditative techniques and for that reason is more properly the subject of a separate book, which I hope to write some day. This chapter is like the preparatory stages of a gourmet meal, where a wonderful aroma is in the air. The volume on advanced sexual meditation, when it eventually appears, will serve as the feast itself.

There are two reasons to read any how-to book about Taoist sexual practices. The first is the satisfaction that stems from finding out about new and useful ideas and perspectives concerning the human condition and spirituality. Sex is, after all, a very popular human activity. The second reason is to actually learn the material.

Sexual energy work can be very powerful. In order for it to be safe and to fulfill the promise of turning sexual activity into something sacred and real, an individual's sensitivity must grow. What are the goals to be working toward when

THE WAY OF LIU
The Master Liu Hung Chieh and Sex

 Liu seemed to be a natural-born celibate. As a youth, he was a staunch Confucian who took his family obligations seriously. He told me that when he was young, his primary motivation for having sex was to have children to fulfill his ancestral obligation, to continue the family line. I asked him, "Did you ever enjoy having sex?" He said he could get through it, but that sex was a nonevent for him. He said that for him practicing calligraphy or martial arts, or reading the various Chinese classics, was a more engrossing experience and significantly more enjoyable and satisfying than having sex. Liu added that being celibate had no particular spiritual advantage.

Liu did point out that asexual people can also valuably use sex to clear out their internal blockages. If a person is naturally asexual, he or she may still have a mildly sexual lifestyle through deeply caring for someone who requires some small amount of sexuality as part of the bonding mix. However, it is important for such asexuals to engage in sex only when both the mind and body naturally turn toward sex. Otherwise, the asexual mind can become distracted during the sex act and meander or undergo visualizations that have nothing to do with the person they are with (that is, the mind may dwell on mathematics or scholarly pondering, or chess, etc.). People with particularly strong personalities are particularly capable of this "uninvolved sex." Even if his lover is the true love of his life–the person who can turn him on beyond all others–the asexual must be turned on by the "idea" of making love in each specific instance, or the act of making love becomes boring.

responsibly learning the more advanced sexual meditative techniques? Here are a few:

1.   Cultivating a genuine respect for the naturalness and sacredness of sexuality. You have risen in a heartfelt way above the sexuality of a base animal, and you have developed all the courage and patience necessary for this challenging and satisfying spiritual task.

2. Doing nothing to your partner you would not want done to yourself. You possess an internal perspective that has already shifted or is shifting toward the idea of a balance between the sexes (rather than remaining mired in the war of the sexes) and toward intimacy and harmonious human sexual relationships, not alienation.

3. Being on the road to feeling and understanding your own and your partner's body. Ideally:
    - You are able to recognize if your own or your partner's sexual nerves are stressed, and can either remedy the situation or accept it without self-recrimination or guilt.
    - Your hands and mouth are highly energetic and sensitive.
    - You are beginning to feel inside the layers of your partner's energy.
    - You are acquiring practical experience of how the energetic genital anatomy zones affect the sexual act, and are beginning to recognize their postcoital chain reactions. This allows you to become aware of how the deeper layers of sexual energy affects your emotions.

4. Getting comfortable with basic foreplay and energy skills:
    - Your hands have a high degree of sensitivity and liveliness, either acquired naturally or from tofu practice.
    - You can energetically feel and manipulate your partner's genitals and sexual energy with relaxed adroitness for at least ten to fifteen minutes. Having refined manual manipulation skills, before beginning the advanced energetics that come into play after penetration, makes a real difference.
    - You have practical experience of being aware of your partner's yin and yang functional energy needs and have developed the patience and

willingness to implement their full energetic possibilities during sex.

- You can dissolve, transfer, push, and pull sex energy around your own body without strain, so you can recognize the nature of sexual energy without it putting you in a hormonal trance or distracting you from being aware of your spiritual essence.

5.   Having at least some ability to use the inner dissolving process, both sitting and during the sexual experience.

- Your partner dissolving exercises involving hand, foot, and head holding should be beginning to bear fruit, both during the exercise and during the enjoyment of sex.
- If your partner is not a practitioner, you should be somewhat able to dissolve both the energies of yourself and your partner during foreplay.
- If both of you are practitioners, you want to reach a level where both of you can link and dissolve the same energy or energies, simultaneously.

Feeling confident within yourself, you may find it interesting to try the more advanced sexual meditative practices. The advanced practices will enhance your understanding of the possibilities of sex in the overall context of human spirituality, especially the energetic potential of human sexuality in terms of meditation.

Internal Alchemy

CHAPTER
8

I Ching Hexagram 15–Humility
Changing line–6 in the second place

A superior man of humility and worth
Takes things all the way to their natural ends

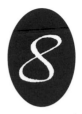

Internal Alchemy

What Is Alchemy?

There were two forms of alchemy in ancient China: external alchemy and internal alchemy, the latter of which we examine in this chapter. When we think of external alchemy, which was also practiced in medieval Europe and the Middle East, we tend to conjure up images of a wizard wearing a black gown and pointed hat, toiling in a sequestered laboratory with flasks, beakers, and burners, trying to turn lead into gold.

When internal alchemy is mentioned, most people don't know what picture to conjure. Some might dredge up an image of a yogi sitting cross-legged in an cave, back straight and eyes closed, working on "enlightenment," or they might envision mystic charts with arcane symbols of energy centers, chakras, and intricate lines representing energy channels. Today, people are doing internal alchemy practices not only in caves and monasteries but also in their homes and apartments, either sitting on the floor or in chairs, using the same concepts of the internal alchemists of old: transmute, change, transfigure, stabilize, and continue.

External alchemists were seeking to create, distill, and magically transmute physical substances, especially herbs, minerals, and metals. Their costly lab experiments were aimed at two great accomplishments: turning lead into gold and creating a physical substance called the "philosopher's stone," which, when ingested, supposedly cured any disease, reversed the aging process, and conferred physical immortality

–the ultimate pill, as it were. The external alchemists were part of a larger mystical tradition. As such, it is mistaken to think of them simply as the precursors of modern chemists. In antiquity, alchemists, internal and external, were held to be wise men with developed souls.

Internal alchemy uses as its laboratory the human body, mind, and consciousness. Consequently, for the internal alchemists the equivalent of changing lead into gold became the changing of their own foolishness into wisdom, greed to generosity, anger into compassion, judgment to equanimity, and fear into acceptance. They didn't seek physical immortality so much as complete freedom for the Consciousness or soul. In Taoist internal alchemy, the alchemical precepts progressed to living in the Tao by means of a series of transformations: body to chi to spirit to emptiness to Tao. Although the term *internal alchemy* may mean different things in different Taoist traditions, the common bond is a series of transformations.

There are many ways to accomplish these transformations. Most are unexplainable in a book as they must be taught by a living adept. A central technique, however, is the dissolving practice that forms the core of this volume. Moreover, there are specific methodologies for each of the eight energy bodies, an exhaustive treatment of which is outside the scope of this book. What is practical here, however, is a more detailed look at how internal alchemy can transform emotions. Transforming the emotions is the most coarse level of alchemy, which is why we may begin here.

Alchemy and Emotions

Emotions are valuable to humans. They give tremendous color to life. Zombies do not seem to have them; robots certainly do not. Human emotions motivate us toward action and are integral to our survival. When our emotions are activated, the energy released from our glands invigorates us physically. All our emotions and internal organs are interlinked, each being part of the energetic cause and ultimate manifestation of the others. Some find strong emotions such as fear and anger to be deeply uncomfortable. Taoist internal alchemy, however perceives the energies of powerful emotions not as something to avoid, but rather as necessary and life affirming, when we distill what is valuable in them.

Every emotion has a yin aspect, a yang aspect, and a nondual or neutral aspect; in other words, we are filled with opposing yin-yang energies, consisting of the useful and the useless, the nectar and the poison, as well as the original neutral source of both these dualities.* Fear and anger are two primary emotions. In the case of fear, the nectar is courage, the neutral aspect is intensified awareness, and the poison is terror or paralysis. In the case of anger, the nectar is compassion, the neutral aspect is the ability to act, and the poison is the destructive impulse.

Energetically, fear awakens the kidneys–the vital center for activating chi throughout all the internal organs, and in turn all the body systems those organs affect. This explains fear's devastating power on humans; chi from the kidneys courses deeply into every nook and cranny of our bodies, it jolts the body awake and keeps the whole body aware. Likewise, anger energetically activates the chi of the liver, the center which motivates our muscles, and primes and maintains our ability to act.

In prehistoric times, when a tiger charged into a cave of humans they needed their fear and anger to survive. Today, when confronted by danger, either real or perceived, we will go through a similar process of fear and anger.

For cave dwellers, the sudden shock of the tiger activated their kidneys, sending a sudden surge of kidney chi throughout their bodies and causing each person to react from one of fear's characteristic aspects. Some could become

*In Chinese, the terms for this are *yin*, *yang*, and *tai chi*. Tai chi is the source of yin and yang and is neither yet both. The slow-motion meditative exercise called tai chi chuan takes its name from this lofty philosophical principle. Tai chi chuan in the Taoist meditation tradition is a practical method of experientially realizing what these words actually mean, by using your own body as the tool for that realization.

sharply aware (the neutral), using the fear to give them the ability to weigh their options, for example, to flee, fight, or trick the tiger. Others could act courageously (the nectar); one person might sacrifice his or her self so the rest of the group could escape. The energy of fear could cause others to become mentally disassociated and unaware–making them unable to see a situation for what it actually was–or they might become petrified into catatonia (the poison).

The poison of fear can be quite harmful beyond the immediate situation that triggers it. If you habitually react with the poison of paralysis, your glands release internal body toxins that damage the kidneys and thus weaken physical health and diminish vitality. You also become predisposed toward releasing the internal body essences that make it easy for you to become depressed.

At a deep soul level, humans are often structurally confined to a narrow range of responses to the energy fear generates. Our conscious awareness of what is useful to do in threatening circumstances can be overridden, causing us to unconsciously react from structures energetically hardwired into our systems. Instinctively, for example, we could fight or flee the tiger, or cower and freeze in terror, rather than working from heightened awareness and possibly astutely tricking it into leaving us alone. The poison may override the neutral or the positive, constricting our ability to adapt rapidly and constructively. Taoists say this constriction is probably due to primal attachments to the physical body and the ego.

As said earlier, with fear often comes anger. The tiger's appearance in the cave would also activate the liver and thereby send a surge of energy to the muscles, giving one strength. Without appropriate powerful anger these early humans probably could not club the tiger with sufficient vigor, yell loud enough at it to scare it off, fight through the pain if it wounded them, or free their stamina to act long enough to deal with the problem. Fear may give you the awareness to perceive what to do, but anger gives you the power to follow through and surmount a seeming impossibility.

Anger's neutral power can easily flow into nectar or poison. Anger's ability to spur you to action can direct some people toward compassion–the nectar. In the ancient Greek tale of Androcles and lion, Androcles courageously and compassionately takes a thorn out of the lion's paw, thereby relieving its pain, and removing the impetus for its crazed terrorizing of the local village. In contrast, others might let their anger turn into an incessant need for violence–the poison. Throwing a rock might scare away the tiger, however they would choose to slay the tiger because they enjoyed the thrill of the kill.

The poison of anger–the incessant need for violence–can hurt you in many ways. It can weaken your liver and dispose you to having an inappropriate temper, which will play havoc with your human relationships and cause unnecessary stress, diminishing your peace of mind.

In a dangerous situation, the ability of fear to heighten your awareness and the ability of anger to motivate you to act are necessary for humans. From one point of view, both are neutral in the sense that being aware or being able to act does not say what form these will take. Some people's natural inclination may be for fear to jolt them from awareness to paralysis; while others might move from awareness to courageous action. Similarly, anger's ability to spur action may naturally steer one person toward harmful deeds and another toward compassionate ones.

The way a person expresses their emotions both verbally and nonverbally (in action) is what we call human demeanor and character. The dissolving process of water method Taoist meditation resolves the obstacles associated with the conditions which helped mold your character after you were conceived and prevent you from recognizing your individual essence that the Taoists call the body of individuality (see Chapter 2 of *Relaxing into Your Being*). The water method of alchemy is concerned with how you can literally change the character you brought into this world, and the way your energy manifests in the world, going beyond the confines of your inbred nature which is based on your genetic (or karmic) structure.

Three Tools of Internal Alchemy: Dissolving, Visualization, and Sound Work

Water method internal alchemy uses both the methodologies of visualization and sound work from the fire traditions and the dissolving techniques from the water traditions. In the water method, once the light of consciousness has been released by one's reaching the Great Stillness, the dangerous aspects of the heat generated by fire methods have been removed. Neither the light inside water nor fire is then hazardous to meditators. The fire techniques of sound and visualization can easily be destabilizing if the fangs of our hidden human dysfunctions are not first rendered harmless by the dissolving method. By the time you reach the state of alchemy in Taoist meditation, the safety features of the water method have been installed. The final goals of alchemy can then be reached by the water method of dissolving alone or by combining it with fire methods.

Dissolving

As emphasized, the dissolving practices employ the focused attention of the heart-mind to break up internal bound energy until that energy becomes neutral and can be reformed for more useful functions, where previously it had congealed into stagnant, less useful shapes or configurations. Nothing is created in this process; rather, whatever is not part of your individual essence falls away, to be reused. The phenomenon is much like that which occurs in modern waste recycling, where used bottles are reduced to liquefied glass to be poured into molds, which can be customized to fit the needs of the moment. The liquid glass has no need to resume its former shape or assume any other future shape.

Visualization

A visualization is different–rather than simply making new bottles from old, it breaks the old bottles down into molecules and reconfigures the molecules into a newly created substance, such as a silicon chip. The visualization provides design specifications for the intentionally created silicon chip–limitations, possibilities, shape, density, and so forth. Using visualization, a person may transform the paralyzing poisons of fear into courage or hope, or the destructive poisons of anger into compassion.

The visualization may be created purely from your focused mental intent, or standardized versions may be used, such as those from Taoist icons, which are the Chinese equivalents of the more familiar Christian icons or Tibetan paintings depicting gods, angels, demons, saints, or Buddhas. Each part of the painting or visualization–the clothing, the facial expression, the body posture–corresponds to specific traits that the meditator wishes to transform using specific techniques–fear into calmness, anger into compassion, greed into kindness, and so on.

Visualization is not merely a matter of turning on a television screen in your brain and seeing disembodied, empty images–a relatively easy exercise for most people in the electronic age. Rather, you must viscerally imagine the event happening, as if it were something that fully engages all of your capacities–a real event for you, not just a meaningless picture. For some people, this visceral feeling will be a more immediate entryway into visualization than mental images. Simultaneously combining seeing and feeling, the visualization first seems to be something outside yourself. Later it becomes your own self, right down to your hair, blood, and bone marrow. Over time, this process will change the quality that the seventh energy body, or body of individuality, emanates. Each desired change requires altering the different components of your visualization, which may zero in on transforming one part of the picture at a time or on the whole picture at once.

With internal alchemy, you refine your character in the same way that the external alchemists refined metal–that is, progressively changing the vibratory level of the metal so it is transformed from lead to various intermediary substances and finally into gold. As with precious stones, many stages are gone through, as a garnet becomes an opal, then a ruby, and then a diamond. Each refinement distills out the impurities that mask your essence. Sometimes the visualization process involves elaborate rituals, but usually not. The Taoists tend to get to the main point quickly, with a minimum of ritualistic preamble.

Sound

Alchemists believe that all phenomena are created from vibrational energy.* Sound, which is one form of vibrational energy, is used in two ways in internal alchemy. The first is similar to the applications of the tantric traditions, which combine the uttering of specific mantras with visualization. (Because Chinese is a tonal language, in which inflection over a range of four to eleven tones can completely alter meaning, the Chinese mantras are exceedingly difficult for most Westerners to learn.) These specific mystical sounds shake up the frequencies of the underlying vibrational structure of your internal "lead" or "zinc" (your spiritual character or emanation), eventually shifting the underlying structure to the new frequency and thus replacing the old. While making the sounds occur, the practitioner puts his or her body in particular postures (either sitting still or moving) that allows the energy to shift frequency most easily. These postures have been worked out through thousands of years of experience.

The second, more complex method of using sound applies controlled frequencies that literally vibrate your insides, energy bodies, energy channels, and visualizations. These oscillating sound patterns are not normally heard in the Western world. They not only have a powerful underlying vibration but also continuously change as they move through an extraordinary range of tones and overtones. This

---

*This concept is echoed in John 1:1: "In the beginning was the Word (that is, vibration), and the Word was with God, and the Word was God."

method allows you to break up an underlying energetic vibrational level, reduce the vibrational pattern to a neutral frequency, and reconfigure that frequency to a new one (lead to zinc), which you deliberately create or allow to come into being. Moving through a wide range of pitches, you use full effort without strain to infuse these sounds with all your intent and the power of Consciousness itself.

Both vibrational sound methods may be done in three different ways:

1. You first make your sounds audibly, with a normal voice, until you can say the sounds smoothly, without freezing up. You then gradually progress to a louder and louder voice, until you are projecting your sound and can be heard a great distance away.* When your voice begins to get stronger, you concentrate on physically vibrating the insides of your body—muscles, soft tissue, skin, internal organs, blood vessels, glands, and bones. After you can do such vibrating *without strain*, you may begin to vibrate certain specific places in the brain.** This process must be done only under the careful guidance of an experienced adept. Once you have begun the process, stopping before you are fully balanced is not wise. You may have unleashed forces for which you are not prepared, and which no one could predict beforehand. These forces need to be fully processed, so you are not left internally dangling. You continue working until you can bring the volume of the sounds from a normal voice to a near yell and back again *easily and without strain*.

---

*To learn how to avoid possible strain of the vocal cords when making loud sounds, consult a singing teacher or voice coach.

**There are thirty distinct centers in the brain that are directly related to the functions of the upper tantien. Traditional Taoist masters restrict the teaching of these centers only to those whom they deem to be prepared for it and for whom they judge it to be safe.

2.   Next, you make the same sounds at a near whisper. Paradoxically, the softer your voice becomes, the stronger the internal vibrations become. The deeper the vibrations go, the more specifically you are able to target them inside your body, and the more powerful the energy becomes. This paradox–the softer the voice, the more powerful and penetrating the energy–can be grasped only through practice. You continue to decrease the volume until the sound becomes silence, at which point your focus is strongest.

3.   Previously, you focused on the overall sense of your energy body, but now you can use your inaudible vibrating to target the exact energy channels that connect to your first six energy bodies. You now focus not only on your emotions but also on the specific internal organs and glands that power the emotions. You then focus on the brain centers linked to those emotions, and then on the energy channels and tantiens that link these centers to every part of each of the seven energy bodies through which they function.* Each shift of vibration changes the totality of the underlying energy field that you emanate in that moment. Another shift stabilizes the energy pattern. Eventually, when you have transformed each of the first six energy bodies separately, you then transform all six into a single fused energy that is joined with the seventh body.

The practices usually begin by working with and fully opening the lower tantien, then the upper tantien and the brain centers. Then the energies of the lower and upper

---

*Although the number of energy channels that empower the first seven bodies totals five thousand, only those who go into the deepest recesses of Taoist energy practice ever need to work with more than twenty of them. This level of expertise is usually reserved for chi gung masters, energetic therapists, and alchemists, and not for the average person or even committed student of Taoism, who would be overwhelmed by such a task.

tantiens are brought into the middle tantien to fully open the heart center. All fuse in the middle tantien, in the center of the heart-mind, creating an awareness of Consciousness beyond mere energetic phenomena.

Visualization, vibration, and sensation all eventually fuse into a united whole to transform what you are working on at the time. As you master all the processes necessary to complete the integration of the energies within your physical body, you will then move out into space to complete the process away from your body, first to the boundary of your etheric (chi) body. Then the same for your emotional body, beyond your etheric body to the stars and outward, farther away from your physical body with each successive energy body, as you become more and more stable in the Consciousness within you, until eventually you transform everything as far as you can go to the ends of a never ending universe.

Sooner or later, a jump in Consciousness spontaneously arises where the underlying structure fully transmutes to Consciousness. The "red dust" becomes Universal Consciousness itself. You will now act from the Tao rather than the human mind. The human being who reaches this stage has become the superior person of the *I Ching* and a guardian of the worlds. This individual has become one with the Tao.

Internal Alchemy and the Recognition of Universal Consciousness

Let's look closely at how internal alchemy works in the water school. In this tradition, alchemy is begun only after a practitioner has meditated to the point where the Great Stillness is achieved. Only after you know what Consciousness itself is are you clear what is water (pure Consciousness) and what is red dust (the contents of Consciousness).

The remaining dust itself is not composed of our basic dysfunctions or past traumas, for these have already been cleared out through dissolving. Often, in many fire methods of Taoism, the term *alchemy* is applied to practices that turn our dysfunctional emotions into nonreactive emotions. In the water tradition, these problems are not part of the alchemy practices; they are, rather, handled by the dissolving practices. Why?

Using the example of gemstones, we need to make a distinction. Old multilayered dirt and residue (the first to the sixth energy bodies) encrusting a gemstone must be differentiated from the gem itself (the seventh energy body, the body of individuality). Garnets, rubies, and diamonds are different types of gems, so each makes a distinctive kind of necklace (each manifests its energy in a different way). In the water method of alchemy, we take great care to distinguish between the innate structure of a human's "red dust" and the true nature that the dust camouflages. The Taoist meditative dissolving process (the pre-alchemy stage) deals with the encrustations. Internal alchemy deals with the intrinsic nature of the gemstone itself.

The goal of internal alchemy is to transmute in stages the underlying structural quality of the gemstone into the water of Universal Consciousness itself. This task cannot even be attempted while people are focused on the need to feel good about what is inside themselves. One must begin from the point of knowing what is inside, without ambiguity, so that when the dust is internally transmuted into water, there will be no doubt that a transmutation has in fact occurred. If you are merely transforming one belief about Consciousness into another belief, you may find yourself on endless mind trips with no change whatsoever happening at your spiritual core.

In some branches of the fire school, the traditional practice is to initially take all the blockages in your first six energy bodies and release them in much the same sequence as the dissolving methods of the water school. The fire method, however, accomplishes this by creating tremendous physical heat in the lower tantien. The purpose of this heat is to incinerate your bound internal blockages. (This process can take a long time, just as the fundamental dissolving methods can.)

As the bulk of the gross traumas, attachments, and so on, are being cleared out, the heat in the lower tantien becomes extremely fierce–enough to cause profuse sweating. Eventually, burned-off gross matter naturally turns into a ball of light and drops down into the perineum, just as, in the water method of meditation, the encrusted material dissolves, leaving only the unadorned gem. From here, the process of internal alchemy called *nei dan* begins. The ball of light commences to circulate throughout the microcosmic orbit. There are specific alchemical procedures for each place where the ball arrives. Gradually, the ball of light links all the energy centers and channels in the body, transmuting them into Consciousness, which then begins to expand, body by body, until it encompasses the whole of the universe.

Some Taoist esoteric schools apply the sound and light transformation techniques right from the beginning, especially at the emotional level. They go directly to changing anger to compassion, fear to awareness, greed to generosity, hatred into joy, and so on. However, they do this without having first released the encrusted material around Consciousness itself. As soon as they build up energy from a chi gung or energy circulation practice, they start transforming emotions without hesitation. Both the water school and many fire schools, such as the one previously described, disagree with this process because of its potential long-term implications.

They agree that it is possible to transform one emotion into another successfully, with tremendous speed. The problem with this way of transformation is that it can permit practitioners not to feel those parts of themselves that are slightly on the dark side. They may only experience their "feel good" side. They now have an effective shield protecting them from feeling or even noticing the potentially cruel, nasty, capricious, supercilious, venal, or unaware parts of themselves. This new power tool relieves them of all this unpleasantness, whose existence they can ignore, blithely believing that all is well with the world. They find their energy increased, yet something remains wrong, seriously wrong, because their deep underlying structure has not changed, only the quality of the encrusted dirt adhering to the surface of the gemstone.

The internal tools of alchemy can be very strong. Using its techniques, your awareness, vitality, and mental acuity can become stronger and your personal power can grow. But consider the gods of ancient Greece. They too were powerful. Through the accident of being born on Mount Olympus, good luck, or mystical ritual practice, they acquired great power. However, beneath it all they had not dealt with the petty stuff of humanity. They could not feel or even care about what the poor mortals who were affected by their power were going through. The Greek gods often behaved like all-powerful infants who granted boons and pleasures but, when they had a tantrum, would inflict great pain and suffering on defenseless humans. For all their powers, they were often egomaniacs who could be devious, capricious, and cruel. They did what they liked, often with no sense of balance, justice, or any semblance of the Golden Rule.

When the psychic side of internal alchemy dawns, anyone can drift into a predicament like that of the Greek gods. If you lose contact with the depth of your own human pains and potential dysfunctions your increased awareness and powers can lead you to a spiritual dead end. The deeper underlying dirt may be worsened, but you won't know, because your surface dirt is made to feel good. Your compassion or awareness will be tainted by your underlying nonsense, but you won't know it. For example, a sadist may shift from overt nastiness to a passive-aggressive's cruel compassion. The Taoists of both the water and many fire schools believe that this condition moves anyone farther away from the Tao.

Self-delusion can be a greater and more powerful enemy to spiritual evolution than a direct desire to be evil. Self-deluded people can cause havoc, yet delude themselves and manipulate others into thinking that they are basically good souls. Evil–the practice of raw power without compassion–will sooner or later show itself unambiguously. Such was the world of the Greek gods. This is why the water school believes that first a student should personally experience the guiding positive reality of Consciousness itself, as an internal living role model, before embarking on the path of internal alchemy.

Stillness and Internal Alchemy

You might ask, where does one find peace in all this complexity of technique? At the completion of each stage of practice, one must arrive at a place where the yin and yang energetic relationship has become balanced and hence comfortable. This harmony results in what the Taoists call *jing*, or stillness, the Consciousness totally unmoving and comfortable with itself. This stillness is the basic framework of all the classical schools of Lao Tse's Taoism. The Taoist word for meditation is *jing dzuo*, which means "to sit in stillness."

At the stage of internal alchemy, you start transmuting the very cells of your body. You actually change your physical capacities, overriding your natural intrinsic limitations. Of necessity, the body now has to be changed into something capable of handling and not distorting the psychic and causal energies involved as well as being able to keep itself from being damaged.

The fundamental principle of alchemy is that things exist in both gross and subtle forms. Is the energy of your Consciousness very condensed, or is it spread out to where it has no boundaries? When you deal with energy inside your body (the chi, your emotions, your mind, the psychic level, or the source inside you from which all of these events spring), you are experiencing different levels of energy condensation. Your natural awareness is squeezed into a straitjacket. As this energy releases (that is, becomes more open), the natural capacity of your mind and body emerges.

THE WAY OF LIU
My First Day of Meditation: Does Meditation Change after You Are Enlightened?

 I learned from Liu that the water tradition of Taoism considers focusing on enlightenment, on the coming to a final victory or endpoint, to be nonsense. The Buddhists speak of "breaking the wheel of reincarnation;" a Gnostic Christian might speak of "becoming one with God." The word Tao means "the way," "the avenue, street, road." Whatever term you want to use, the point is that, in Taoism, things really do not have a beginning or end. There is no brass ring at the end of the journey. There is no "I got it," no "aha!" It would probably be nice if such were the case, but Taoism is not amenable to accomplishing that. There is no big deal about the experience of enlightenment; it is, rather, about living from that place, without fuss, bother, or exaggeration.

After being with Liu for a while, I began to notice that my internal world was becoming easier to coexist with, as though I had gained or accomplished something and somehow became stronger. I fantasized about what it would be like to be free of all of life's burdens after acquiring "it." I asked Liu outright what life would be like after "enlightenment."

Liu said, "At various levels before enlightenment much of my life was wishes, hopes, fears, and all kinds of beliefs about what should and should not be. Afterward, things were just what they were, no more and no less. I still breathed, ate, and defecated as before. I meditated every day for years before the event and have every day since. Not much has changed, except that before I was yearning to understand how to meditate well and afterward I knew how to do it. Meditation is not about obtaining a magical external accomplishment, it's about living a full life in harmony with your inner and outer world. The red dust of the world is always landing on and obscuring the clarity of one's mind. After enlightenment, meditating simply allows you to polish your mind, continuously removing the newly accumulating red dust and keeping your consciousness clean, clear, and pristine."

When I began my own first day of meditation, Liu said to me, "I simply became enlightened my first day of meditation, and I have continued to meditate regularly since." He told me I could relax my anxiety or hopes about enlightenment, as I was meditating now and would continue to do so after enlightenment. "Nothing much," Liu said, "will change."

The Taoists hold that there is as much "space" inside of you as there is in the infinite external universe. The mind can travel the same distance inward as it can outward in the universe. In one sense, developing more energy is about the capacity to let those energies that can go out, go out–and for that matter, it is to let those energies that can go in, go in, as far as it is possible to condense inward.

Once you start to become involved in Taoist alchemy the presumption has been made that you have already completed the practices of becoming a mature human being.

As you go deeper and deeper into meditation, you simply get involved in the essential nature of how things are. Stillness in essence and practical function become the guideposts when you start doing internal alchemy. You begin yet again working with the channels of the body. You begin transforming the quality of the essences and energies themselves. You again work with the energy of the environment, the sun and the stars, the earth, the five elements. You begin transmuting the various levels of emptiness you encounter. But when you sincerely start working on these things, you find out that probably the most difficult part is having to take responsibility for every single individual action you take internally as well as in the external activities of the world, the "red dust." From here on, you really begin to focus on the middle and upper tantiens.

There begins strong investigation into understanding the essential nature of the universe, how manifestation occurs, and how the intrinsic nature of love permeates these manifestations. This is the work of the heart center (the middle tantien), which has to do with relationships–of yourself to others, to living things, to the earth, to the stars, to your Consciousness itself. The heart practice in Taoism is exceedingly strong stuff.

In advanced alchemy, one also becomes involved with the upper-tantien practices (the thirty energy centers in the brain), which have to do with time and space, and literally going beyond time and space. As you start getting into the upper-tantien practices, you start becoming aware that there is more going on than what is just here on earth. You discover that everything you do, although it is unimportant because it does not exist long in the grand scheme of things, nevertheless has profound temporary effects at the level of Chi.

You start having to take responsibility for your actions. Almost everyone learns this lesson the hard way. You start finding out about human limitations. Your spirit does not have a limitation, but your body and mind definitely do.

Your work with the three tantiens, with the channels of energy in the body, and with the states of mind that go with them, becomes of critical importance. Now, in the process of transforming the physicality of the body into spirit and moving the energies, something starts happening to your physical body. The cells start changing. You don't end up with the body of a normal human being. Your body starts molding into what your mind really wants. You gradually learn the genuine relationships between what is and is not conscious, the ultimate objective being to make all eight of your energy bodies fully, not partially, conscious.

The Taoist water method tends to be much softer than other methods of meditation. Yet one must not confuse softness with weakness. A tidal wave is plenty strong. The whole method of letting everything just come together, with full effort and yet no strain, is a hallmark of the Taoist water tradition.

The work in getting from spirit to emptiness is fun; it's wild, interesting, intense. When one genuinely gets involved in meditation, it is a twenty-four-hour-a-day involvement. You have now made the decision to fully engage your life. Once you do that, ultimately you will be spiritually fine. You will also learn a few lessons along the way, both pleasant and unpleasant. Taking the bitter with the sweet goes with the territory.

It is a long struggle, but at the end of the long road of alchemy, you become one with the Tao.

Back to Balance

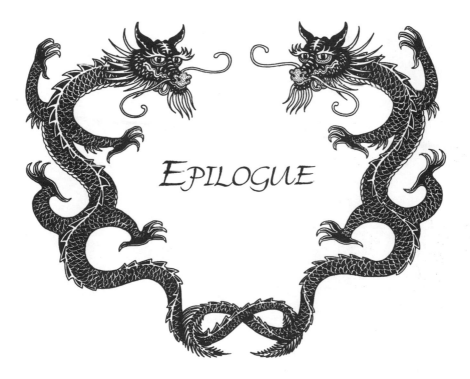

EPILOGUE

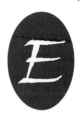

Back to Balance

This book has covered a lot of material. At its conclusion, it is fitting to refer to Taoism's central theme: balance–balance in our body, energy, and emotions, in our hearts and minds, and between our innermost essence and the Tao, the spiritual root of the universe.

In this era, life speeds along faster than it ever has before and changes quickly in ways that we neither completely understand nor feel we have the ability to control. Often the traditional spiritual and secular foundations of our lives no longer seem relevant. Anxiety, uneasiness, or discomfort are constantly present in our inner world. It is becoming exceedingly difficult to remain calm and to cope in a whirlwind world of stress where traditional values regarding work, free time, family, and spirituality are being tossed aside.

This book has tried to show some ways to bring personal balance back into your life. All the exercises in this book are geared toward increasing your inner awareness. At every juncture of your day-to-day living, you can use that awareness to look at how you are living and interacting with life. Practicing the breathing exercises at the end of Chapter 1, and in the first volume of this series, *Relaxing into Your Being*, can soften and relax your mind and body at any time, especially when the pressure is on. Bringing the energies of your body into equilibrium can enable your mind to balance all the inputs coming into your perception, whether or not you begin with your mental gears screeching or running smoothly as if oiled.

Practicing the 70 percent rule progressively creates balance in anyone who follows it. The 70 percent rule is the foundation of the water method of meditation. It can be summed up in three simple related statements:

1.   Do not do too much or too little.
2.   Use your full effort without strain.
3.   Be gentle with yourself, without internally collapsing or beating yourself up.

Achieving balance has always been difficult and is now virtually a lost art. The progressive path of water method meditation allows for the kind of self-reflection necessary for internal balance to be reborn and nourished. Each stage of the water method practice further enables individuals to develop balance within themselves and in their interactions with events and living beings, friend and foe alike. The preparatory practices harmonize your body and the energies that make your body work. The intermediate practices balance your emotions, mental processes, and psychic perceptions, and help you to genuinely comprehend that what people sow, so truly do they reap. Finally, the advanced alchemical practices bring you into balance with the forces of the universe and the Tao.

Being aware of the possibilities inherent in internal alchemy can keep returning you to seek an authentic source of living spiritual inspiration: Universal Consciousness itself. The sheer human act of searching for Consciousness, both within yourself and, eventually, in everything all around you, generates balance in all its forms. The quest for something larger than your own self tends to bring out the twins–balance and compassion. In the midst of the hustle bustle, the panic, the overdue deadline, it is good to realize that we can change the patterns of our life, bit by bit, if only we sometimes try.

The mind and body are locked in many chicken-and-egg structures. For one example, the deeper structure of the mind influences the way you hold your body, and your body posture affects your thoughts, emotions, and judgments. The five styles of Taoist meditation practice bring balance to your body posture (however it is formed) and to the flowing chi energy of your body, enhancing your health. While physically balancing your body, you can simultaneously focus your awareness on balancing your thoughts and perceptions. This focus requires just little extra effort as you stand, move, sit, lie down, or engage in sexual contact.

As you practice specific techniques or simply observe daily situations, it will be natural for you to notice what internally blocks you from allowing balance to manifest in your being. By using the inner dissolving approach, you can dissolve these internal obstacles that unbalance the emotional, mental, psychic, and causal aspects of your inner being. As more and more of these obstacles dissolve and resolve, leaving no shadow, glimpses of Consciousness will flicker through your awareness. Dissolving deeper and deeper inside will also progressively free you from the psychic tensions that prevent you from relaxing into your being.

Balancing human relationships, and sexual relationships in particular, is and has always been tricky. Taoist sexual meditation offers a different and far greater vision of sexual intimacy than is usual. It discusses ways of bringing harmony rather than hostility to sexual relations. Knowledge of how to energetically help balance what is bound in your sexual partner (an advanced practice) and helping to release his or her deep psychic tensions is a distinct contribution the Taoists have made to humanity. The tofu and other basic sensitivity exercises presented in this book, which enhance the physical and basic energetic aspects of sex, are the beginning steps toward such balance.

If you conscientiously work with meditation, attaining a degree of stillness naturally brings forth balance in your body, mind, and spirit. Manifesting any level of stillness and emptiness in your mind empowers you to catch a glimpse of, and reunite with, the Consciousness that is present inside you and all around you. This awareness is a fine first step in bringing forth the inner light that is within us all. The sheer act of coming into contact with Consciousness tends to move the human mind toward recognizing balance.

The good news is that balance can be found if you sincerely seek it. The other news is that unfortunately, in many challenging situations, finding balance is neither easy nor simple. If, as the Taoists believe, all life in this universe is seamlessly interconnected in an endless spiritual web, then finding ways to balance whatever parts of the web each of us personally influences is one of life's greatest challenges.

We cannot always easily change the external world. Well-intentioned mass political and social solutions often produce cures that are worse than the original disease. Throughout the ages, the Taoists saw that the real cures for societal ills reside in changing the innermost spiritual hearts of people, one by one. For without the wisdom born of balance, human choices made from goodwill often turn out to be foolish and of no avail.

Taoists believe that if balance could be nurtured in enough individuals, the seeds for a better future society would be sown. Balanced human beings are more likely to be interested in and capable of producing balanced, sustainable societies and environments. Out-of-balance, emotionally unresolved people usually maintain societies based on greed, shortsightedness, and lack of humanity. Taoists observed that, especially in dark times, only the emergence of genuine spirituality can bring back the balance necessary to prevent mankind's natural tendencies toward destructive human folly.

Daily practice of Taoist meditation can be compared to the actions of a single raindrop landing in a reservoir. Just as single raindrops fill a reservoir, daily attempts at bringing balance into your life gradually fill your reservoir of clarity, creativity, and common sense. Eventually, each individual's reservoir of balance can spill over and beneficially influence the ocean of humanity, creating the compassion and wisdom necessary to catalyze real change during critical historical times. In this way, what we do with our inner lives matters in our daily lives and for the planet as an interconnected whole.

Sitting in a Chair
for Meditation

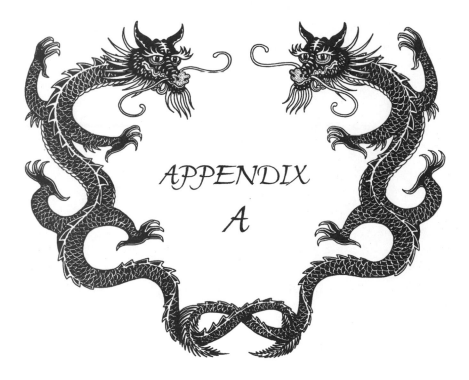

APPENDIX

A

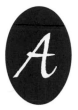

Sitting in a Chair for Meditation

The Mechanism of the Problem

The problem of pain brought about by prolonged sitting in a chair, whether in meditation or working at a desk, is caused by the progressive contraction and shortening of the deep muscles and fascia from the bottom of the pelvis to the navel. If this contraction of the thighs, hips, and belly is strong enough, the strain will extend higher, and all the soft tissue between your head and your pelvis will be pulled downward. The longer you sit, the more the contracting originating in your pelvis will tighten and bring fatigue to the muscles, tendons, and vertebrae all the way up to your neck and shoulders, with the potential to cause any one of them to misalign. Contraction in your muscles, in turn, can overstretch your ligaments, stressing your hip and knee joints, causing pain.

The solution lies in stretching out the deep muscles and soft tissue (ligaments, tendons, and fasciae*) from your knee to your kwa and lower belly at any time those tissues begin to shorten or fatigue **(Fig. 11)**. You accomplish this stretching by making small movements of your pelvis and trunk during sitting. These movements reestablish the nerve signals to the offending muscles, instructing them to keep stretched and not collapse, thus preventing pain and fatigue.

*A fascia (pl. *fasciae*) is a sheet of connective tissue covering or binding together internal body structures.

Figure 11 Deep Muscles of the Kwa

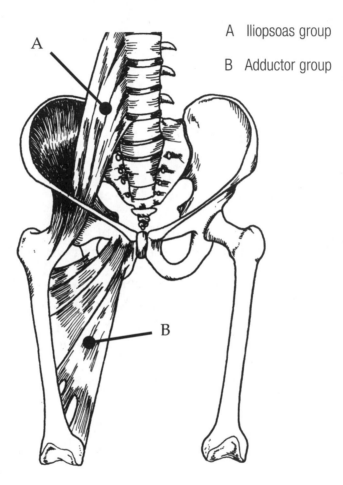

A   Iliopsoas group

B   Adductor group

Illustration reprinted from *Opening the Energy Gates of Your Body*

The trick is to maintain the spring of the soft tissues inside the kwa, by eliminating slack or involuntary contractions, and yet avoid becoming too taut.

To understand this mechanism more fully, think of these muscles and other soft tissues inside your body as a series of interconnected rubber bands. You want to make sure that during any period of prolonged sitting (whether in meditation, recreation, or office work) that the even, continuous tension that allows the "rubber bands" to exert maximum elasticity and strength is maintained. It is the function of the soft tissue to hold your body up, and not the function of your bones, as most people think. These "rubber bands," which bear the weight of your body, are connected to each other. If one of them becomes overly slack, it causes another to become overly taut, pulling in turn on a third. For example, if the pull between the knees and back is excessive, other muscles can overstretch and pull out tendons, ligaments, and vertebrae; also, your knee and hip sockets can become misaligned.

Another way to conceive the situation of your muscles, soft tissues, and joints as you sit is to imagine your soft tissue as a cloth ribbon. A length of fabric can be even and smooth, or it can have creases. If your body tissues are like smooth cloth (that is, creaseless), you normally will not experience physical pain or unnecessary fatigue. Creases, however, will ordinarily bring pain and long-term chronic damage, especially when they snap open and close shut again at odd angles. If the cloth is allowed too much slack, it will crumple and crease. If pulled too tight, it may tear somewhere (in the body, cartilage, muscle, or ligaments might tear, for example).

Now consider the one continuous piece of cloth as being composed from bottom to top of a spectrum of three colors seamlessly sewn together. The first color band runs from your knee to the inguinal fold at your hip.

The second color band is what we have identified as the kwa. The kwa regulates the energy in the left and right energy channels of the body.* As you can see in **Figure 11**, the kwa contains the iliopsoas muscles. One branch begins from the inguinal cut and the floor of the pelvis and continues up to the top of the hip bones, deep inside the pelvis. The other

---

*A detailed discussion of the kwa, including exercises for gaining control of the iliopsoas muscle group, may be found in B. K. Frantzis, *Opening the Energy Gates of Your Body*, Chapters 5 and 9. (Berkeley, Calif.: North Atlantic Books, 1993).

branch is from the thigh bone (femur) to the lower spine. If the soft tissues of the kwa are pulled more than they should be, they negatively affect the lower back and hips.

The third color band comprises the deep muscles of the midriff, the *internal obliques*, located between the crest of the hip bones and the bottom of the ribs, and the continuation of the iliopsoas muscle to the diaphragm.

Each of these three color bands affects the other. It is necessary to be aware of each independently, as well as their relation to each other. Let's say the uncreased cloth is twenty inches long, with its top and bottom fixed in space (as are the insertion points of your body). If you made a crease of one or two inches in the middle of the cloth, you could cause another part of the cloth to be on the verge of tearing (which is quite painful) or actually tear, causing chronic injury to your knees or hips. If the cloth is not held fixed in space and just sags, it can cause the vertebrae to compress and put pressure on nerves inside the body, resulting in both pain and fatigue. When you hit the fatigue point, you have several choices: live with the pain, which can be distracting at best and physically incapacitating at worst, or restretch your body to its natural length, as if you were taking the creases out of the cloth.

The Solution: Lift, Stretch, and Do Not Close the Kwa

Figures 11.1a and **11.1b** show how the pelvis stretches upward when the kwa opens and collapses when the kwa closes. Opening the kwa is like taking the creases out of the cloth, and closing it is like bringing the creases back. Check that your kwa is open when you begin to sit, and make a special point of checking this at regular intervals. To open your kwa, lift everything you can feel, from your perineum through your pelvis to the top of your hip bones, and then continue feeling a lift through your midriff to the bottom of your ribs, all without lifting your chest. When you accomplish this opening maneuver, the inguinal fold between the top of your leg and the top of your pelvis will straighten out (that is, its crease will flatten out), relieving pain and reducing fatigue. The opposite happens if your kwa closes down and its fold increases–you experience pain and fatigue.

The kwa must be gently lifted and not forced, as it causes the most powerful pressure on your body's "length of cloth." Make sure this gentle lift slowly stretches the soft tissue to your knees and shoulders, so that neither feels pulled or painful. Also, do not deliberately contract your anus as you lift the kwa. The anus will be lifted effortlessly by the kwa action itself.

Figures 11.1a and 11.1b Lifting the Kwa

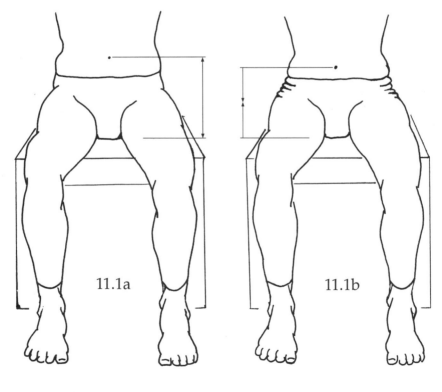

11a Correct position: 11b Incorrect position:
     the kwa open and lifted   the kwa closed down

Exercises to Stretch the Kwa While Sitting in a Chair

To alleviate the discomfort of prolonged sitting, most people move their shoulders, which does little to help the lower back. The four exercises described here, however, not only help the lower back but also release painful pressure on your shoulders. When the kwa begins to weaken or close, the following four exercises can effectively return the body to an uncreased state.

The following suggestions will help you achieve the ideal posture to maintain throughout your sitting meditation:

- Gently press your feet continuously into the ground throughout each exercise to obtain a solid connection from your feet to your spine. Press until your knees feel quite stable, without any slipping or wobbling.
- Extend and elongate your muscles upward from your knees to and through your kwa, all the way up to your lowest ribs. If done well, this stretching will noticeably release the muscles of your lower, middle, and upper back, as well as your shoulders and neck, without your deliberately moving them. Depending on your size and the original amount of contraction in your kwa, your body could lengthen anywhere from half an inch to three inches. The better you become at mentally relinquishing the contraction of your nerves, the bigger the stretch and release of the torso.

When you feel your body beginning the slippery slide to ever-worsening contraction, or you feel your mind weakening and becoming distracted, you can use these four exercises. (Begin with the simpler external movements of exercises 1 and 2.) The exercises are all performed in the same way and yield the same benefits when used for meditation whether sitting in a chair or on the floor. In all these exercises, your hands should remain in your choice of one of the three palm positions described in Chapter 3 (see p. 77).

Exercise 1

1. Continuously keep your spine absolutely straight (without hunching your back) from your tailbone to the top of your head.

2. Bend forward from your inguinal fold and return to your original starting point slowly and rhythmically so that you gradually restretch your kwa and midriff. In general, the bend will usually be in the range of 6 to 18 inches. Use the 70 percent rule as a guideline to know how far to stretch forward without exceeding your limits. If you are in the process of meditating, bend only as far as you can both comfortably maintain your internal work and relieve your body of distracting pain. If you use this exercise to relieve the pain that can come from desk work at the office, you may want to pause from work for a moment and put your full attention on rehabilitating your back. Your increase in productivity will more than compensate for the time lost. Remember, this movement is in the long-term interest of your back.

3. *Maintaining the straight spine* described in step 1, stretch your kwa and midriff by moving your body in a circle, as follows. First lean your whole spine slightly forward, then to the right, then slightly back, then to the left, and then forward again, using the center of your pelvis as the center of your circle. As you execute this circling, it is important to extend continuously from your perineum through the center of your body up the front of your spine and out from the top of your head. Pay particular attention to stretching from the knee through the kwa and midriff when you get to the left and right sides of the circle. Do your best to even out any imbalance on either side by moving more slowly or extending higher on the more contracted side. Pay extra attention to lifting

the kwa when moving through the sides of the circle.

4.   Next, repeating steps 1-3, make a second circle moving your body in the opposite direction in order to balance out your small internal stretches.

Exercise 2

1.   Bend your spine slightly forward by focusing on releasing your vertebrae from their posterior (back) side, one by one, beginning from your tailbone and progressively moving upward to the top of your neck **(Figs. 12a–d)**.

2.   Raise the vertebrae of your spine by focusing on pushing up from deep inside your belly and the anterior (front) side of your vertebrae, one by one, again beginning from your tailbone to the top of your head **(Figs. 12.1e–h)**.

Figure 12 The Sitting Spine Stretch, First Half

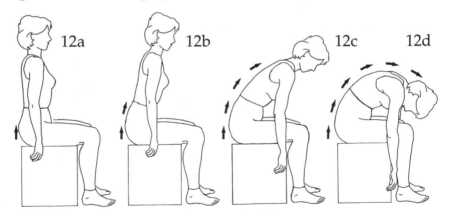

12a   Starting posture: back straight, head lifted, chest dropped, belly relaxed, shoulders rounded.

12b–d Gradually release vertebrae from bottom to top, bending forward as each release is achieved. Release from the posterior (back) side of the vertebrae.

3.　　If one side of your body is more contracted than
the other, place more emphasis on pushing up the
kwa on the side that is near the contraction–that is,
if your left side is more contracted, use more effort
for the kwa on the left side than for the kwa on the
right side.*

Two advanced techniques–kwa pulsing and pumping
the spinal fluid–are also important to sitting meditation but
are beyond the scope of this book. The internal work necessary to do both techniques are taught as part of the author's
six-part chi gung program (see p. 270). This program teaches

Figure 12.1 The Sitting Spine Stretch, Second Half

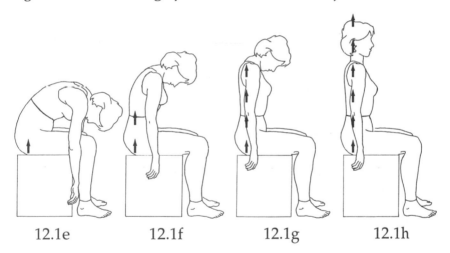

　　12.1e　　　　　12.1f　　　　　12.1g　　　　　12.1h

12e　　Posture upon completion of first half (you are bent all the way
　　　　forward).

12f–h　As you sit up straight, open the anterior (front) side of the spine
　　　　from bottom to top. Opening means lifting each vertebra in the
　　　　front (vertebrae are already opened in back from the first part of
　　　　the stretch).

*The steps in exercise 2, which is executed in a sitting posture, are the same as
those of the tai chi spinal stretch, which is executed in a standing posture. The
complete details of the standing spinal stretch may be found in B. K. Frantzis,
Opening the Energy Gates of Your Body, Chapter 10 (Berkeley, Calif.: North
Atlantic Books, 1993).

the 16 components of Taoist nei gung (see Chapter 2 of *Relaxing into Your Being.*

When the kwa begins to crease, keep your spine, neck, and head straight and still. Without moving forward, to the sides, or backward, do the following two exercises, which are more internal.

Exercise 3

Gently open and close* (increase and decrease the distance between) both the kwa and midriff. This movement will cause the spaces between the lower lumbar vertebrae to pulse, creating more distance between the vertebrae and removing misalignments in the lower lumbar vertebrae.

It is important that the pumping of the kwa and midriff be very gentle, not sudden or sharp. From your knee to your midriff, all of your soft tissue must move evenly, each section in proportion to the others, without one section exceeding or lagging behind another. Pump only as far as the tightest part of your soft tissue can go (that is, to its "weakest link"), from the knee to the bottom of your ribs. For example, if the upper part of your thighs can internally move only a very little but your kwa can move a lot, reduce the movement of your kwa to match the more restricted movement of your thighs. Once all the tissues are equally stretched and are moving evenly, pump only to a maximum of 70 percent of their potential range of motion.

Once you have taken out all of the micro-creases in your lower body you will find that you can sit fairly effortlessly for very long periods of time.

Exercise 4

This exercise, which uses a full spinal pump,** is a physical technique used for opening and controlling the

---

*These openings and closings are part of the author's *Marriage of Heaven and Earth* chi gung program (see p. 271).

**The spinal pump is taught in the author's spinal chi gung program, *Bend the Bow and Shoot the Arrow* (see p. 271).

body's major energy channels, as well as for circulating energy throughout the body. When the spine pumps, it evenly and proportionately stretches and pumps all the body's tissues, the complete ribbon of cloth. The whole length of our internal elastic rubber band (that is, the soft tissues: muscles, fascia, tendons, and ligaments) is pulled apart and comes closer together, evenly and without breaks, thereby stimulating the spaces between the vertebrae, the bones of the skull, the joints, the cavities, the soft tissues, the internal organs, and eventually, the brain and glands. This method can be targeted to allow you to pump and reset only one or two misaligned vertebrae.

Should One Foot Be in Front of the Other?

When sitting in a chair, it is ideal to have the tips of your toes equally forward as if touching the same line, with feet parallel and the middle of each foot aligned with your left and right energy channels. Over time, gently try to over-come any tendency you might have to splay your feet apart. (If there is pain involved for you in this, let your feet remain splayed as little as possible.) The backs of both knees should feel slightly and equally stretched rather than contracted.

If one side of your body is significantly more creased and contracted than the other, it is valuable when you are internally lengthening your body to put the foot of the more contracted side forward. This foot position will stretch the contracted side more than the side that is loose. After both sides become evenly stretched, you can bring both feet even with each other again. If you cannot tell which side is contracted, have a friend observe you and indicate if one part of your body looks uneven or contorted. Contortions are caused by contractions.

Sitting on the Floor
for Meditation

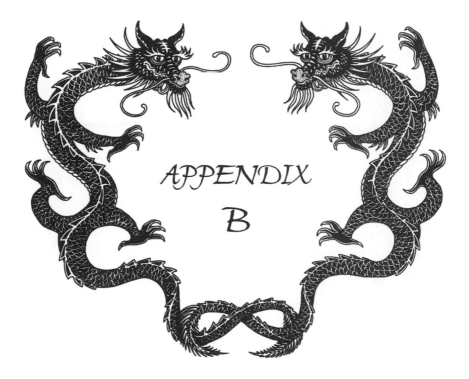

APPENDIX

B

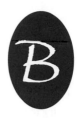

Sitting on the Floor for Meditation

Before you sit on the floor for Taoist meditation, review the body alignments for sitting in a chair (pp. 76–9). Remember, you do not have to sit with your legs twisted like an Indian yogi to meditate—not everyone can sit for long in a cross-legged position without running the risk of knee damage. For those whose bodies are loose enough to sit comfortably on the floor unsupported (with or without a cushion) the following points will be helpful.

What Causes Knee Pain during Prolonged Cross-Legged Sitting on the Floor?

It is the norm in Western cultures to sit in chairs rather than on floors, as people in China or India do. Consequently, most adult Westerners, having been reared in "chair cultures," need plenty of practice to do protracted cross-legged sitting on the floor to meditate. The cross-legged position strains the back, hips, and knees significantly more than does sitting in a chair. In addition, most people in the West are unused to the flat-footed squatting posture used routinely in other cultures. Flat-footed squatting stretches the muscles related to the hip, knee and psoas to their natural potential, which is required for prolonged painless sitting with a straight back. Loose, elastic soft muscles promote strong blood circulation, thus reducing body pain, whereas hard, inelastic contracted muscles reduce blood circulation, causing increased body pain, especially in the lower back and legs. Babies can sit with a straight back effortlessly because their psoas and leg muscles are both stretched and soft. Most Western adults cannot because their psoas and leg muscles have become both shortened and hard. Such over-contracting can lead to the lower body's ligaments and muscles being progressively pulled out from their insertion points, resulting in pain, joint damage, or both.

The longer that cross-legged meditators sit, the more their circulation weakens. This weakening causes the muscles to contract and shrinkage to occur in the space between the pelvic bones, hip sockets, knee, and ankle joints, which further blocks circulation, which further shrinks the muscles in an ever-increasing, painful destructive spiral. This nasty downward cycle works in this manner: Tight midriff muscles pull the psoas muscles, which pull inelastic thigh muscles, which pull, overstrain, and possibly tear the liga-ments that hold the knee together, misaligning the knee joint and, over time, possibly damaging the cartilage, bringing long-term chronic knee pain. In the process, the upper buttock muscles (gluteus maximus) contract, as may the lower back muscles, possibly causing the lower lumbar vertebrae to go painfully out of alignment.

At this point, pain or numbness in the lower back, leg muscles, knees, or hips will either force the cross-legged meditator to stop, endure excruciating pain, or become temporarily (or perhaps chronically) injured. The older a person is, the worse the situation usually becomes. Many of those whose strategy for pain is to "tough it out" exceed their bodies' limitations. Often, the next day, they have to see their chiropractor, acupuncturist, or massage therapist for pain relief. If individuals push too far, they run the risk of severely tearing the anterior cruciate ligament, necessitating a visit to a surgeon skilled in microsurgery.

The solution to this serious problem is to release and lengthen the midriff, psoas, thigh, and knee muscles fully. Whether sitting with or without a cushion, *you should only* bend your knees further or go lower once they are completely comfortable and feel no strain at all.* This principle will allow you to remove all excessive pressure on the knee. Learning how to follow it requires awareness, relaxation, and patience.

Releasing to Stretch a Muscle Is Different from Pushing to Stretch a Muscle

It is important for you to relax, let go, and release your legs, rather than try to push and stretch them further. Many people attempting to extend their legs into a progressively stretched sitting position get goal-obsessed and willfully stretch their legs and knees further than their body can comfortably go. Use of force often results in a severe back-lash—your muscles will badly tighten up over the next week. By relaxing the legs and letting go into the stretch, you can more easily feel subtle pains, those early warning signs that ligaments or tendons arc becoming overstrained. When people overexert to attain a full lotus posture, the long-term knee problems that ensue usually come not from muscle damage but from ligament damage, which is the worst kind. The "letting go" method repatterns (that is, teaches) your central nervous system to react to stress and strain with a relaxation response rather than habitual tension.

From the Ming Men Point, Simultaneously Open Your Body Equally Up and Down to Protect Your Knees, Hips, and Lower Back

Relax and open your whole body, so you gradually get a sense of creating space inside your body rather than feeling your body shrink and contract. Emphasize opening

*In addition to traditional belts that wrap around the lower body, giving support to the lower back and knees, newer high-tech belts can do an even better job. These lightweight belts often enable a person who could sit for only five minutes before pain sets in to sit comfortably for over an hour. For many, such belts are a good intermediate step to sitting in the classic cross-legged way.

your pelvic area, especially increasing the space in and around your hip sockets, sit bones, and perineum. Let the felt distance inside your body from your lower back through your hip sockets, knees, ankles, and feet increase, so you feel like your legs, and most importantly your knees, are opening up away from your hip socket and lower spine.

Use the ming men point (see *Relaxing into Your Being*, p. 164) on your lower back as a starting midpoint. Release equally up and down your body from that midpoint. As you release from the ming men point, simultaneously extend your lower back and legs downward, while at the same time you equally release, stretch, and extend your spine upward. For example, if you open half an inch upward in increments, you also open half an inch downward in equal increments. In order to release your spine, deeply relax both the back and neck muscles and relax and get a sense of space deep inside your belly, chest, and throat. The more you wish your spine to go upward, the more your chest should soften and release downward. Relaxation, a sense of space inside the torso, and physically creating space in between the spinal vertebrae and joints needs to be done gradually and progressively without force when you practice cross-legged sitting.

Do Not Force the Knees to Bend or Drop; Rather, Release from the Kwa and Hip Sockets to Protect your Knee Ligaments

If you, like most Westerners, did not grow up sitting on the floor, when first sitting cross-legged you should not put one foot on top of the other thigh. Instead, initially cross your legs at the ankles or shins, with your feet as far away from the pelvis as necessary for you to be completely comfortable. Over time, gradually bring your crossed feet toward your perineum. You should move your crossed feet in stages of no more than one inch per week or month, or even more time depending on how stiff you are, in order to avoid stretching the knee ligaments too rapidly. Bringing the feet in toward the pelvis too swiftly can cause unnecessary pain and can damage the ligaments by diminishing your ability, either immediately or in the future, to hold your knee joint stably in place.

First, using the dissolving process, bring about a deep release in your pelvis and a relaxation of your back muscles before you move your feet closer to your torso or attempt to lower your knees. Most stiff-legged people, in their overzealousness, try to push down and stretch the knee first, a dangerous practice that can lead to knee problems. For the safety of your knee ligaments, it is important that your pelvis, hip socket, and kwa release first, stretching the muscles and fascia down to your knee gently, before attempting to stretch the knee itself.

In cross-legged sitting, your feet need to be comfortably stabilized at no more than three or four inches from your pelvis (ideally, touching your pelvis) before you attempt to put one foot on top of the other thigh. It is not required for anyone to use a half or full lotus position in order to meditate. If you want to assume either of these positions, however, you must completely release the inside of the pelvis *first* before your knee fully drops down or you put your foot higher up the opposite thigh toward your hip socket. Remember that in terms of releasing your nerves and stretching your soft tissue, first release the inside of your pelvis (hip sockets and kwa) and midriff; next release and stretch the thigh muscles; and lastly, minimally stretch the knee. *You want any strain to be taken by your kwa and hips, not your knees.*

If you do put one foot on top of the other thigh, make sure you are absolutely comfortable, without any strain inside your kwa and hip joints, before attempting to bring your feet the next half-inch closer to your pelvic bones.

Should the Left or Right Leg Be on Top?

Many, if not most, people have one side of their body tighter or looser than the other. These left/right body imbalances manifest during cross-legged sitting either because the chi is significantly stronger or weaker on one side or because the body's tissues on the left or the right are significantly more contracted or stretched. Such conditions frequently exist in or around one or more of the following areas: internal organs, midriff, ribs, kwa, hips and buttocks, thighs, or calves. These left/right body imbalances are usually caused by bad posture, shortened or twisted muscles, previous physical or emotional illness or traumas, chronic tension, back problems, or blocked energy channels.

If your kwa is blocked on one side or the other, it usually indicates a blockage in the left or right energy channel of your body. Such blocking can inhibit you from using the energy from the earth to your advantage. It can also effectively cut your body's energy in half at the waist, inhibiting your lower tantien from fully storing chi. If the earth energy component is not fully available to your body, you are stopped from successfully completing many of the five-element chi practices of Taoism. Energetic blockage in the legs also prevents the complete circulation and transference of energy up and down the body and from side to side, which is required in many intermediate Taoist meditation techniques. Most Westerners find moving energy in the upper body to be much easier than moving energy in the legs.

In general, when sitting cross-legged, remember that you want to simultaneously stretch your internal creases (see Appendix A) equally and evenly, upward and downward, inch by inch, from your lower tantien. You also want to adapt the four kwa-stretching exercises for sitting in a chair (also in Appendix A) to sitting on the floor.

When you sit in a cross-legged position, there are several situations that determine which leg to put on top of the opposite thigh, for how long, and how to get your knee completely down.

1.   *Both of your legs are more or less evenly stretched*
If your legs are balanced, then simply switch which leg is
on top, either when you get to about 70 percent of your
fatigue point or when you know the strain is beginning a
slippery slope to becoming too painful. Always adhere to
this 70 percent rule (that is, never exceed 70 percent of your
capacity), which applies to all Taoist practices, including
sitting. Make sure that you let both your knees go down to
an equal distance from the ground before switching leg
positions. If your body is loose enough that you do not
need to change leg positions during a given meditation
session, then alternate which leg is on top at every other
practice session. Correct any left/right leg imbalances *before*
you ever begin using this method of alternating legs.

2.   *One of your legs is only marginally tighter than the other*
Maintain the 70 percent rule when switching from one leg
to the other. Spend a little more than half of your practice
time with your tighter leg on top, thereby stretching it out
more. Do this until both knees drop completely down, fully
relaxed and evenly stretched. You should practice until your
hips feel completely relaxed, without any internal pulling or
strain present.

3.   *One of your legs is radically tighter, with its knee*
         significantly higher than your other knee
Most people naturally tend to avoid pain and put their
looser leg in the difficult position (that is, on top of the
opposite thigh). Although this may work in the beginning,
over time it will cause your tighter leg to become even more
contracted and out of balance, ultimately making the tighter
leg worse and potentially damaging it and rendering you
unable to sit for prolonged periods on the floor. The thicker
a person's legs, the worse the problem can become.

        One useful strategy for alleviating this negative situa-
tion is, for a short period only, to first place your looser leg
forward or on top until the pelvic nerves relax, release, and
your leg drops a bit. At this point there will be some residual
nerve transference to the opposite leg and the tighter side
will have stretched a little, beginning the relaxation response.

Next, switch your tighter leg into the more difficult position. When you again hit your 70 percent pain threshold, bring your looser leg back to the more difficult position and keep it there until you get the relaxation response again and your tighter leg releases. Keep repeating the leg-switching cycle.

If your tighter leg is on top of the looser thigh, with its knee up in the air, and you get a big release that causes the knee to drop substantially, stay in the dropped knee position for no more than a minute. Then take your foot off your thigh and put your foot down and in front of you in a new, less-strained position. Often, when a tight leg releases suddenly, immediately afterward the body will snap back like a rubber band and, at the level of the nerves, reinstitute the contraction response. By putting your foot on the floor, you allow your pelvic nerves to complete their release, preventing the counterforce that can, in a time-released fashion, overstrain the knees. Stay sitting with the just-released leg in front until the nerves of your hips fully release and your legs and hips feel comfortable and stable.

Sitting on a Cushion on the Floor

Many meditators sit on cushions, elevating their hips some distance from their knees on the floor. They sit in this manner to lessen the strain of gravity pulling on their hips and legs while simultaneously maintaining a strong, stable sitting posture. Before you lower your hips closer to the ground through removing blankets or substituting a smaller cushion, make sure that both the up and down stretchings of your legs and your spine have reached their full, uncontracted, comfortable length at your previous height before going lower. This cautionary step will mean not removing more than a half-inch of padding each step down, until you are eventually sitting flat on the floor. It is best to stretch your lower body only 70 percent as much as you think you are capable. Doing so creates an essential margin of safety.

Frequently Asked Questions about Taoist Meditation

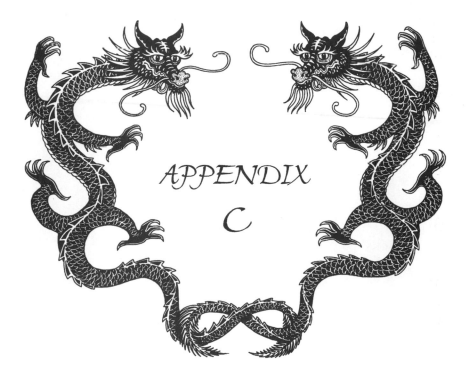

APPENDIX

C

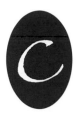

Frequently Asked Questions about Taoist Meditation

1. Are chakras and tantiens the same?

Not exactly, although both terms denote major energy centers of the human body. The seven chakras of the yogic system (or nine, if you count the chakras above the head) are primarily the gateways to different levels of human consciousness. They only tangentially influence human physical health, through psychological and psychic inter-links. The three tantiens of the Chinese system are also gate-ways to the different levels of human consciousness. However, the lower tantien also directly controls all the energy channels, both major and minor, which govern and regulate all aspects of physical health.

Trying to understand the similarities and differences between both systems intellectually is an immensely complex task. From all sorts of functional points of view, key points of both the tantien and chakra systems are sometimes the same, sometimes similar, and sometimes completely different. It is best, at least initially, to study each system entirely on its own terms. After you have experientially stud-ied both systems equally in depth, the connections and inter-links between them will become obvious.

2. Some emotions seem to throw up great barriers to being dissolved. Is this a sign that I need to focus on them or a sign that I should leave them alone?

This is a personal decision. However, remember the basic meditation dissolving principle: if you feel as if you will spend five minutes or five thousand years dissolving something without any resolution, move on to the next emotional blockage or sensation to be dissolved. The roots of the emotion will not go away. You may though, need to resolve some different but interconnected secondary energies that are holding the main emotional block in place. This secondary work has to be accomplished before you can naturally return to the original emotional energy for a complete resolution or gain access to the next deeper layer of this specific emotional onion. Toughing it out may or may not bring an emotion to an earlier resolution. Rather, the act of staying too long on something that will not resolve can cause you to travel in circles and create unnecessary work. This is because the time has not yet arrived. When the time arrives, enough auxiliary energies will have been released or softened; that is, those energies that previously have formed a brake on completely resolving the central emotional issue. By the same token, however, do not just leave dissolving an emotion alone because it is discomforting or you wish to avoid dealing with it.

Regarding emotions and the inner dissolving process, the central question essentially boils down to, What is too much or too little? Learning this balance point, which is as fine as a razor's edge, is a major challenge for every serious meditator. While teachers of the water method of Taoist meditation can offer guidance, learning this balance is an art that each meditator must ultimately find for himself or herself. The application of common sense to your inner world is central to all sincere and eventually successful meditators' basic requirement of taking responsibility for themselves.

3. How do I keep from falling asleep during seated meditation?

This problem is and has always been a major one for meditators. You are not singled out if it happens to you. If you are sleep deprived, which is a rampant condition in modern society and one that causes many accidents, it is probably best to get some rest or actual sleep before you meditate. Realize that the state of meditation is basically akin to that experienced right before actually dozing off in real life. The mind slows, so it is important to realize that you must do things to stay awake just as you would if you were falling asleep but needed to keep alert to complete a task.

Maintaining proper body alignments can help a great deal to prevent you from falling asleep. Incorrect alignments cause your energy channels to close down, which de-energizes your body and overloads your nerves, making you dull and sleepy, whether or not you were initially tired or fully awake and rested. Pay particular attention to straightening your spine and to lifting your midriff and occiput at regular intervals.

Get used to practicing the standing and moving modes first before engaging in the more difficult sitting practices. It is harder to fall asleep standing up or moving. The standing and moving modes are an easier training ground than sitting for learning to stay awake and deeply relax, to stay aware of your insides where you can begin to notice the mindstream.

Excessive carbon dioxide in the bloodstream will tend to put you to sleep. Sitting meditation will cause the inside of your body and brain to work hard, consume a lot of oxygen, and produce carbon dioxide. If you meditate while sitting and your breath is shallow and weak, carbon dioxide can build up, causing drowsiness. If you begin to doze, breathe deeply! If that isn't sufficient, try this simple breathing exercise that, if done for three or more breaths taking less than a minute, can expel the excess carbon dioxide from your system, thus re-energizing your nerves and keeping you

244 The Great Stillness

awake: First, deeply inhale through your nose only. Next, exhale from your mouth using four to six "machine gun" explosive breaths in rapid succession, until *all* the air is out of your lungs. This rapidly releases the carbon dioxide.

The image of a sitting person falling gently asleep is more or less a cultural stereotype. A person falling asleep when sitting and reading a book, for example, is not at all unusual. If you have learned any tricks in life to keep sleep away in this situation, apply them when you feel yourself nodding off in meditation.

4. Are there any kinds of guideposts that indicate if the inner dissolving process is working for me?

The best guidepost is a simple before-and-after contrast. Where were you internally before you applied the inner dissolving process on something specific? Where were you internally after dissolving? Is the sting the same, less, or different? Have you dissolved and gone past one more layer of your negative emotional onion and become aware of what is really underneath your initial emotional reaction? After focusing for some days, weeks, or months, are you moving toward resolution of a lifelong problem, or at least finding that you can now live with it, without it tearing up your insides? Does the dissolving process help you to reach equanimity with what before was always an unresolvable and highly charged set of feelings inside you? Are you beginning to change?

As a beginner, target a specific negative emotion or emotional pattern, dissolve it, and personally experience what the difference is. First find something that perpetually gets your negative emotions going, reflexively. There are so many: a memory of a perceived wrong done to you, a political position you cannot abide, something you are immensely jealous of, something that makes your greed salivate, a person or group you hate, a deep regret, a painful memory that will not leave, or an unresolved hangover from your relationship with your parents, lovers, friends, enemies, and so on. Second, focus on dissolving the obstacles that keep you from generating any positive state you may want to establish: the ability to be tolerant, to love, to accept love, to live without fear, and so forth.

Gradually you will build enough experience to be able to discover internally whether dissolving has in fact occurred, or whether you have only shifted the same piece of content from one place on your internal board to another, without substantially changing anything at all. Of course, the more subtle the content you are working on, the greater your sensitivity will need to be in order to realistically discriminate between definable internal landmarks in this very subjective area. Conversely, the grosser or more violent the emotions you are dealing with, the easier it will be to gauge whether something is happening or not.

Another guidepost for testing yourself occurs when a real-life situation naturally surfaces. One of my students, a thirty-eight-year-old male massage practitioner in Phoenix, Arizona, was involved in a passionate love affair, which was to him the most physically and emotionally satisfying relationship of his life. One day, the love of his life declared she didn't want to see him for a while and was going back to her boyfriend of thirteen years. He became enraged, a common emotional reaction to rejection. He even considered going to his girlfriend's office and tearing it apart, instigating a disruptive spurned lover's scene.

Realizing that this could create a mess, he stood and practiced dissolving. After some minutes, his rage naturally led him to his liver, the internal organ directly associated with anger. During a long dissolving session, he dissolved inward and outward, away from his liver. Gradually his seething passed and did not return. This surprised him, being contrary to the way his emotional life had worked before. The next day he awoke calm, exhibiting some of the physical symptoms that normally accompany detoxification of the liver.

Questions Reprinted from *Relaxing into Your Being*

1. In the standing and moving practices, how do you deal with the mental and physical strain than can come from maintaining the required body alignments?

By practicing consistently and applying the 70 percent rule. At each stage of practice, you fluctuate between releasing nerve tension, releasing your habitually shortened small muscles, and stabilizing your mind, all without straining past your limits. Habitual tension fatigues your nerves and shortens your muscles. Tension that has taken decades to harden like cement in your body will take time to dissipate.

Habitual tension, which virtually everyone in our technological society suffers from, weakens the stamina of the nerves that inform your body parts how to maintain proper physical alignment in order to maximize the energy flows in your channels. When your nerves are tired and you force them to perform beyond their capacity, you feel the result as strain and pain. In the many important small muscles needed to comfortably maintain proper physical alignments, cumulative habitual tension within the nerves induces permanent muscular contractions, both overt and subtle. Acquired over years, these habitual contractions shorten the natural length of the small muscles, as well as their associated ligaments and tendons. Shortened muscles add to the aches and pains of maintaining the alignments, as your body is being asked to stretch beyond its current ability in a manner similar to the strain that comes from being forced to do a leg split. Shortened muscles are also responsible for back, neck, and shoulder pain, nearly an epidemic in modern cultures.

The vicious downward spiral goes like this: tension activates the nerves, which signal the muscles to contract, which further shortens the muscles, pulling on the insertion points where they attach to bones and ligaments, which causes fatigue and strain, which causes blood circulation to diminish in the area, which blocks the chi in your energy channels. The blocked chi causes pain, which causes more tension, and the whole downward spiral continuously repeats, ad infinitum.

Now let's look at two necessary activities that can reverse the situation: Achieving softness allows the muscles to stretch and the nerves to release, and therefore lessens tension. Achieving relaxation without collapsing yields softness and a mind that is stable and comfortable with a certain degree of physical stretch, as well as increasing nerve strength so that the nerves can maintain a smooth flow of energy.

Softness comes from lengthening your habitually contracted shortened muscles and tendons. Relaxation comes from mentally letting go of habitual tension in the nerves, by means of the dissolving process. When the nerves relax, their stamina and strength increase. You need strong nerves to be able to tell your muscles to continuously and gently lengthen in the necessary ways. Nerve strength, not muscular strength, is required for you to be able to remain upright. Weight lifters, gymnasts, and others of immense muscular strength have the same problems maintaining soft relaxed alignments as do nonmuscular types. Nerve relaxation causes your muscles to relax. Once deep relaxation occurs, the weight of these soft tissues and associated fluids (that is, blood, lymph, and so on) will gradually and gently pull on your other soft tissues, including ligaments, tendons, and especially fascia. This gentle pulling without tension gradually stretches soft tissues and thereby lengthens them.

Large stretching movements are effective on big muscles but not the tiny muscles that are bound up with fascia. While a bound piece of fascia is in the process of stretching to its natural length, you may feel discomfort or strain. The fascia and shortened muscles and tendons will stretch in increments, with plateaus that need time to be traversed before advancing to the next increment. They will not stretch out instantaneously. If they were forced to, they would be likely to tear.

How quickly nerves will relax and subsequently strengthen, as well as how rapidly your shortened muscles will stretch, cannot be predicted; it depends on each individual. All of us have differing genetic makeups and varying degrees of sensitivity and talent in connecting with internal subtle sensations. The presence or absence of trauma can also affect the rate of the process. What can be said for sure is that the more you regularly do the preliminary practices following the 70 percent rule, the faster the results, and vice versa.

Therefore, you must find your own personal balance between (a) mentally and emotionally letting go of the tension in your nerves, and (b) letting your soft tissues stretch to the new next stage (for example, while lifting your spine or your midriff or dropping your chest). When you have reached a new level, stay there for however many days it takes for your mind to stabilize. Until you have attained stabilization and comfort, do not attempt to stretch even a tiny bit more. It is this trying to go the little bit more–breaking the 70 percent rule–that results in the strain and stress. The tension resulting from the strain in turn prevents the body and mind from relaxing and softening.

Once one alignment has become stabilized and easy for you to achieve without concentration, you may then add another, so that you are doing two different alignments simultaneously. Follow the same procedure until the two are stabilized, then add a third, doing all three at the same time, and so on. Again, the importance of stabilizing at each stage before adding something new must be emphasized. As the chain of alignments you have mastered grows, you may find that an earlier link was not as stable as you thought. Return and rebuild the weak link by again releasing the nerves, restretching the shortened tissue, and stabilizing the mind. Then rebuild the entire chain, from the beginning, without weak links, all over again. If all the other links were solid, this rebuilding process should take only a few seconds, or at most minutes. If another weak link appears, work on it with the same procedure before moving forward.

The point of balance lies in not putting expectations on yourself that exceed your natural limits in the pursuit of perfection. Going beyond your limits ultimately leads to "three steps forward and two steps back," an undesirable approach. Slow and steady is what wins this race.

2. Is it dangerous to practice water method meditation while using prescription drugs?

The prescription drugs of allopathic medicine, along with herbal or homeopathic remedies, are normally used to ameliorate some kind of disease. To the best of my knowledge, practicing Taoist meditation while taking any of these medicines is safe insofar as physiologically based problems are concerned. Taoist meditation has for millennia been used to restore health or to enhance the medical procedures of massage, acupuncture, and bone setting and the herbal remedies found in traditional Chinese medicine. This tradition continues in China today, as hospitals apply tai chi, chi gung, and methods of meditation to a great variety of physical problems. In these hospitals, both traditional Chinese medicine and Western allopathic medicine, including drugs and surgery, complement each other and are integrated to obtain maximum benefit for the patient.

The experience in China has been that the water methods of meditation, being sufficiently gentle, are safe; however, there are cautions, such as in the case of drug-specific dangers from a substance that can lower or raise blood pressure. To be absolutely certain, consult your physician. If dangers exist in the fire methods of Taoist meditation they are generally to be found in excessively forceful practices that encourage cathartic vibrating or intense body shaking, holding of the breath, or muscular contractions.

The question of the impact on one's mental health is another story. I know of no in-depth research or experience to indicate how combining any method of meditation with drugs used for mental illnesses would affect someone with a mental disorder. Tai chi, however, has been used positively to treat the post-traumatic stress disorders of Vietnam veterans.

3. Is it dangerous to practice water method meditation while on recreational drugs?

Taoists believe that recreational drugs dull clarity of mind and thereby retard or completely block progress toward the deeper levels of meditation. True, you can point to a large variety of cultures worldwide that have employed any number of mind-altering drugs to enter into psychic realms. Some of these drugs are integral parts of solid spiritual traditions, but are not part of the water method of Taoism, which purely uses the five modes of practice (standing, moving, sitting, lying down and during sex) without external support.

Having said that, there are some things to consider. We live in a world where drugs are rampant, including alcohol and tobacco. Many who use one drug or another also meditate. A Taoist would typically look at this reality and ponder the practical ramifications involved.

Many young people try recreational drugs to experience the "something more" that they feel is inside themselves but to which they have no access. The use of hallucinogens, for example, often provides the drug taker an expanded internal experience of the possibilities of the body-mind. Such mind/spirit expansions are potentially good, but exploring them with drugs may extract a terrible price. Drug-induced visions, moreover, are not even a remote shadow of what the spirit and Consciousness have to offer a human being.

Once drug users learn through Taoist meditation to go inside and find the living spiritual root that dwells there (however slowly they do this, as the drugs will impede their progress), they just might reduce their intake or perhaps even stop using drugs altogether.

The prolonged use of recreational drugs does indeed retard progress in meditation on many fronts. Taoists in southwestern and western China have always been familiar with all forms of cannabis, as they have lived and live now in regions bordered by Laos, Vietnam, and Pakistan. They found that these substances damage the kidneys and liver and lodge resin residues in the bones of the forehead, residues that slowly leach into the brain, with undesirable results. These side effects distort the energy of the body, slowing the energetic interactions of body, chi, and spirit, which are essential to the Taoist meditation process. Some hallucinogens appear to damage brain functions, a serious obstacle to achieving internal clarity for the meditator, as well as a detriment to obtaining meditative visions, which are clouded by these drugs.

The preparatory practices of meditation can, to some degree, help the alcoholic, the abuser of drugs, and the addict. Throughout history, many chi gung and tai chi masters who practiced long hours daily were alcoholics or opium addicts. Nonetheless, they still managed to retain exceptionally high performance into old age. Normally, alcoholism and addiction to opiates weakens and destroys the body. However, the counterbalancing force of chi practices enabled these chi adepts to withstand the ravages of the toxins they had ingested. Consequently, while still feeling all the anguish that comes from addiction, these masters managed to minimize the damage done to the body through their practices.

The Taoists view addicts as people whose inner worlds are acutely uncomfortable and who take drugs to ease or avoid gnawing psychic or psychological pain. If a person who uses drugs begins to glimpse Consciousness itself, which is part of a meditator's normal spiritual growth curve, a new and satisfying internal environment may take hold. The sense of well-being and wonder at experiencing Consciousness itself may make the effect of drugs pale by comparison. In its pure form, Taoist water method meditation or any other authentic spiritual practice may get a human being higher than any drug.* All that is required is generous portions of patience and practice.

---

*Drug addiction experts and therapists may want to explore the possible use of Taoist meditation's inner and outer dissolving practices as an adjunct therapy within a complete rehabilitation program to help individuals overcome the emotional and mental causes of drug addiction.

4. Does the water method affect one's dreams?

Possibly. There seem to be two basic types of dreams. The first continues or completes internal or external events that occur during the day. The second type involves premonitions of future events, which often but not always come to pass.*

Many things affect the body, mind, and spirit during the course of a day. Most get resolved, some do not. The mind continues to process everything–feelings, perceptions, projections–always seeking resolutions. The problems you may be working on, your hopes, fears, and alternatives, are all played out in dreams. Whole schools of psychological thought attempt to interpret these dreams; whether they are successful or not is a matter of varying opinion.

When meditators practice the inner dissolving meditations, they may release memories deeply buried at the energetic level. In sleep, these memories frequently surface as dreams. The dream itself may resolve the memories or possibly just keep the internal pressure going, so that when you meditate the next day, you can delve into the essence of the dream at a much faster speed and attain resolution earlier than if the dreams had not occurred. Often when memories, including those of "past lives," are released from one's psychic body, the dreams themselves can be particularly vivid, either in color or black and white. These dreams will often indicate normally ignored avenues that you need to work on in your future meditations.

Predictive dreams are more rare. When practitioners work with the psychic and causal bodies, intentionally or not, they may when dreaming see visions of the future. If the tie is to the causal level, the dreams will be very specific and not vague, whereas symbolic visions are usually generated at the emotional or psychic level.

---

*Although part of some Taoist fire traditions, the water school does not have an active tradition of lucid dreaming or of being taught in dreams by non-corporeal teachers.

Liu Hung Chieh was not someone who regularly remembered his dreams. The four vivid dreams he did recall, however, were all predictive. For example, he dreamed clearly the night before he was to take a river cruise on the Yangtse River not to get on a ship. He didn't. Shortly thereafter, the ship sank, killing all on board. Liu did not normally consent to seriously teach students. The only reason he taught me was that on two separate occasions, years apart, he dreamed that he should teach a foreigner who resembled me. On each occasion, without notice, I arrived on his doorstep within the week.

Often, those who do not normally dream will, while sitting and meditating with their eyes open or closed, have visions made of the same stuff of dreams. From the Taoist meditation perspective, as well as those of many other traditions, there exists a continuum between waking reality and the dream state, making it hard to say what is real and what is a dream. A famous story from Chuang Tse concerns a man wondering if an experience was a dream or reality. He muses, "Was I a man dreaming I was a butterfly, or am I a butterfly dreaming I am a man?"

5. Are blockages in the physical body necessarily manifested in the chi and emotional bodies?

Blockages in the physical body are usually reflected in the chi body, but may or may not be manifested in the emotional or other higher bodies. The power that causes your physical body to work is your chi body. A distortion in your physical body will cause some distortion in your chi body, but not necessarily of equal magnitude. The distortion in your physical body could be small and its counterpart in your chi body large, or vice versa.

All this influence is based on the hierarchy of energetic relationships governing the eight bodies (see Chapter 2 of *Relaxing into Your Being*). The blockages or charges in the next higher body or bodies always move downward to affect the lower bodies. In contrast, any lower body has a much more restricted ability to affect the bodies above it. In general, two energetic bodies that border each other (for example, physical-chi, psychic-causal, emotional-mental) are directly linked.

What is influencing what and to what extent, however, is not always so easy to determine. The energy of a blockage as it moves upward from a lower body will always have an effect on the next higher body to some extent, but it will often have little or no effect two or three bodies above. Therefore, disturbance in the physical body may or may not affect the emotional body, and the emotional body may or may not affect the higher causal body, but the emotional body will definitely influence the mental body, and the yet higher psychic body will most definitely affect all bodies below it (mental, emotional, chi, and physical bodies).

Getting a physical bruise will affect your energy body, but may not create a blockage in your emotions or intellectual processes. But a serious blockage in your emotions or way of thinking will sooner or later affect your physical body.

6. What is the difference between quiet chi and agitated chi?

Quiet chi has a sense of smoothness that, when experienced, takes the individual ever more strongly into stillness. Agitated chi vibrates, often very strongly, in a discomforting manner that feels thoroughly wrong, or at the very least not quite right, to people without their knowing why. Agitated chi is one of the overt sources of the "monkey mind." The experience of the sensations of agitated chi may be subtle or rough.

7. How does the 70 percent rule apply to the mind and meditation?

Several common Western maxims carry some of the basic flavor of the 70 percent rule: "moderation in all things," "be gentle with yourself," "appreciate the fact that you have human limitations as well as possibilities," "common sense is good sense," "Rome was not built in a day," and so on.

Some of the attitudes that will cause you to violate the 70 percent rule in meditation are: "self-torture is necessary for spiritual growth," "no pain, no gain," "be perfect or die trying," "grin and bear it even though you know in your heart of hearts that you are going over the edge and will get hurt." While these approaches prevail in most of the world's fire traditions, including those of Taoism, such attitudes are not part of the Taoist water method tradition.

You may have certain expectations about meditation based on what you have read or heard. It is not necessary to pressure yourself. You have to find your own balance point, one that prevents you from psychologically beating yourself up because you feel you are not progressing fast enough. Try to achieve a realistic sense of self-confidence. Don't push too hard and don't be too lazy. In meditation, people exceed the 70 percent rule when they try to be more than human. Gods may be perfect, but not humans. If you are pressuring yourself to be perfect, you most probably are about to throw the 70 percent rule out the window. In meditation, the natural desire to transform yourself spiritually is a good thing. However, this positive desire must be tempered by moderation and an acceptance that going beyond your limits, or forsaking moderation, will prevent you from reaching your goal.

When people first start meditating and going inside themselves, they often have unrealistic expectations of how much sustained pressure their nervous systems and underlying emotions can handle. Consequently, those meditators who push the envelope can destabilize, or "melt down." In regular life, the school of hard knocks trains most of us to recognize the signs that we are beginning to go over the edge. Such signs include agitation unconnected to any present life event, emotional responses that are out of proportion to simple situations, and a pervading sense of physical uneasiness when alone. If signals like these start popping up in your meditation practice, chances are good that they mean the same thing they ordinarily do: you are approaching or going over the edge. The solution: ease off, practice less, or stop for a while. If emotions are arising inside you that you do not know how to handle, *slow down*. It also may be a good idea to seek temporary support from a qualified professional who may have some good advice, or ask a meditation master for insights.

8. How often do I have to keep dissolving before it really works? Twice a day? What do you suggest?

"Before it really works?" This is similar to two virtually unanswerable questions commonly posed by neophyte meditators, namely: "How long will it take me to become spiritual?" and "How long will it take me to become enlightened?" Any individual's ability to progress in any form of meditation depends strongly on your particular karmic makeup and on the kind and quantity of internal obstacles present. Progress in meditation is not linked directly to time spent in practice. What can be said is that if some work is not done on your internal obstacles, they will remain.

When people buy a product–goods or a service–they have a reasonable right to query what expectations the product is going to fulfill, in what period of time. But meditation is not a product. However much or little you practice, it only gives you an opportunity to gain access to yourself–it does not give a guarantee. Practicing sometimes is better than not practicing at all; practicing regularly every day is better than practicing irregularly; practicing twice a day gives you more access than practicing once a day. Sometimes taking a few days or weeks alone or in a group as a meditation retreat, away from the distractions of worldly life, is also very good. In the great meditation traditions of the world, many have been known to take retreats that last for years on end.

9. Does the ability to dissolve diminish with age?

No. Usually the ability to dissolve increases with experience. In Taoism, the dissolving process is taken up quite actively by people fifty or sixty or older.

10. What should the sequence of dissolving be? Do I have to start at the top of my head and always work down, or can I begin at my kneecap and work down from there?

Beginners should always work downward only, and they should start scanning with awareness either at the top of the head or above the head at the boundary of the etheric body. Let's say you have begun moving downward and have reached your chest. If for some reason you now decide to move higher up your body (to your forehead, perhaps) because something is especially bothering you, you must redissolve again everything from your forehead to your chest before redissolving lower down your body toward either your lower tantien or feet.

Do not begin your dissolving below your head, even though the offending energy to which your mind is drawn may be located lower down your body (in your knee, for instance). Clearing what is above the main discomforting blockage, then the blockage itself, and then what is below it is required to release the blockage fully. Often when you are dissolving below your head, the source of the problem will have been resolved before you reach your knee, and when you get to your knee, the initially felt blockage is gone and no longer can be felt. This is similar to acupuncture, where putting a needle in the ear can relieve a kidney problem, whereas putting a needle at the kidney alone may not relieve the organ at all. Similarly, any problem you encounter in your body may not be completely resolved until your awareness reaches your feet. The energetic matrix of the human body is like a hologram, where all the parts are directly linked to some degree or another. Even for an adept, trying to second-guess differing levels of energetic primacy is difficult.

The methodology of the downward-dissolving process was designed to cover all contingencies.

11. Can dissolving occur automatically without my will being involved?

Yes. In the Christian tradition, this is called grace. Grace occurs all on its own without human intervention. Usually, for the beginning meditator the will, or conscious intent, must first be used. After significant experience, rather than after philosophical musings or mere casual experience, the need to use the conscious will can be progressively replaced by a willingness to let things go when you perceive their time has past. If you can't yet let go effortlessly, using intent during the dissolving process will still be necessary.

12. Will inner and outer dissolving work for men and women equally?

Yes. There are natural differences between men and women, of course. Consequently, the genders will initially be drawn to dissolving different aspects of their internal environment. Each sex will find some things easier or more difficult to dissolve than others.

13. Can I dissolve an upper and lower spot simultaneously?

This practice is definitely not recommended for beginners. *Only the downward-dissolving practice is advised for beginners.* Simultaneously dissolving two spots is a fairly advanced practice that requires significant familiarity with the mindstream, which forms the linkage between your mundane conscious awareness and Consciousness itself. Other more advanced dissolving practices include dissolving upward, simultaneously inward and outward, center to periphery, and between entities.

14. Is there a difference between dissolving an emotion or anything else or deciding to ignore it by the force of will?

Yes. Ignoring, suppressing, and dissolving an emotion are entirely different things. As children having to mature into adults needing reasonably harmonious social interactions, we all need to learn some basic emotional self-control. Without it, we would all rip each other's throats out psychologically or physically, without reflecting on it.

However, after you move beyond this basic need for self-control, there is a major difference between ignoring or suppressing a deeply embedded emotion and resolving it. The purpose of the dissolving process is to dissolve and resolve, cut the root of the problem, and finish it, not merely to control it or allow yourself to feel better about it. You must gradually reduce the bound energy until its root is resolved, layer by layer, into Consciousness itself.

When you simply ignore or suppress an emotion, its energy is held in your mind/body and festers, sometimes gradually building to an explosive force, much like the pressure gathering in a volcano before it blows. The buildup is often extremely uncomfortable to live with, both for yourself and others. The dissolving process seeks to release the pressure a little at a time until the blocked emotional energies are dissolved back into their original source, Consciousness itself.

15. Can I use the dissolving process to get rid of things on my skin like warts and blemishes, or deeper internal problems?

I don't know. I can't say I have ever seen anyone try. However, one of my students from Britain relayed to me an interesting incident involving the dissolving experience and his skin. One summer he stepped on a wasp's nest, which shook him up. The angry wasps swarmed and stung him all over his body. He then began to dissolve where he felt the pain most intensely, deciding not to dissolve his calves, which did not feel as bad. Within several hours the considerable physical pain had vanished, and he was calm, no longer emotionally agitated. The next day, the only place in his body that had any pain from the stings were his calves, which he did not dissolve.

In China for thousands of years both chi gung and Taoist meditation also used the dissolving process to heal serious problems inside the body. Once a pregnant student asked me if fibroids could be dissolved, as during her first trimester she developed an extremely large set of fibroids, which were currently growing. After tests the doctors told her that the fibroids had already developed into a large solid mass that would definitely block the birth canal, making a cesarean section necessary. She wanted a natural birth. I said that during my time in China gynecological problems were not my focus as a chi gung therapist, and as such I had no direct experience with fibroids. However, diligent use of the dissolving process has been known to work with other physical problems. I suggested she try, but I offered no guarantees.

She tried. Several months later her hard work paid off. Tests showed that the fibroids had liquefied sufficiently to allow a natural birth. As fate would have it, however, she ended up having a cesarean birth anyway–not because of the fibroids, but because the baby was in breech position. She is currently the mother of a healthy baby girl.

16. Can the dissolving process be done while I have earphones on listening to music?

Not really. In the beginning especially, your undivided attention is absolutely required. Once you become adept at it, you should be equally able to dissolve in the middle of the most horrific or pleasurable situation or noise. Of course, many forms of music are relaxing and emotionally uplifting. Music can take you out of yourself and the incessant problems of life. If you want to go deeper inside yourself and find Consciousness, however, silence is a better complement to meditation than music. Although both music and meditation can tend to put you into a more satisfying emotional space, meditation will eventually enable you to get directly to the heart space without any external vehicles, such as music, art, or other people.

17. Is there any advantage to dissolving in one modality over the other?

Not really. The five modes simply include all the situations life will put you in: that is, standing, moving, sitting, lying down, and relating sexually. Whether one part of life is more advantageous, is better or worse, than another is a matter of personal philosophy. What can be said is that some modalities are easier than others for learning the dissolving process. The outer dissolving process is most easily learned standing. The inner dissolving process is most easily learned sitting. The most difficult way to learn both inner and outer dissolving is lying down.

Energy Anatomy of the Human Body

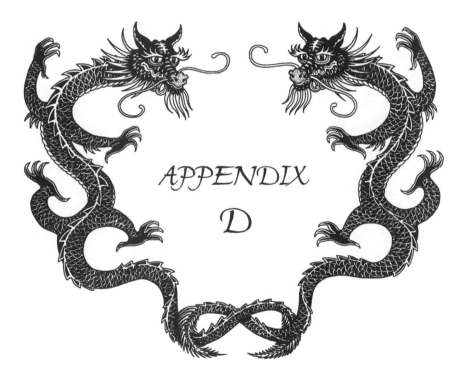

APPENDIX

D

Reprinted from *The Power of Internal Martial Arts*

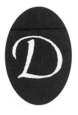

Energy Anatomy of the Human Body

The Main Energy Channels and the Three Tantiens

What Is Common to the Left, Right, and Central Energy Channels

Three main energy channels, or paths of flow—the left, right, and central channels (see Figures 1 and 2)—begin at conception and remain within a person throughout life. Other important energies move in the human body according to meridian patterns that have been well mapped by Chinese medicine. Any text on acupuncture should include charts that identify them. The left, right, and central channels, however, according to Taoist chi gung theory, come into existence before the acupuncture meridians and create these meridians during fetal evelopment. The three main energy channels have certain characteristics in common.

All three, for example, are located in the center of the body; that is, in each, the energy flows occur midway between the skin in the front of the body and the skin in the back of the body.

Also, the central channel joins the right channel on the right side of the body and the left channel on the left side at the tips of the fingers, the tips of the toes, the center of the armpits, kwa, and at the *ba hui* point, which is located on the center of the crown of the head.

The Pathway of the Central Channel

In the torso and head: The central channel runs from the center of the perineum (the area between the anus and the posterior part of the external genitalia) through the center of the torso to the bai hui point on the center of the crown of the head. The channel runs through internal organs, soft tissues, blood vessels, and the brain.

In the arms: The central channel runs from the heart center (middle tantien) to a meeting point in the center of the armpits, where the energies of the central and left or right channels temporarily join. From the armpits, the energy of the central channel moves through the bone marrow of the arm bones, through the center of the elbows and then the wrist joints to the center of the palms and from there, via the bone marrow, to the fingertips. In the fingertips, the energies of the right and left channels on their respective sides merge with the energy of the central channel and, once joined, continue to the edge of the etheric body.

In the legs: The central channel runs through the bone marrow from the perineum between the legs along a line continuing across the pelvis to the kwa and hip sockets. From there it travels through the bone marrow of the leg bones, through the knee and ankle joints, then through the center of each foot along a midline from the heel to the ball of the foot and then through the bone marrow of the toes.

Where the central channel exits the body: The energy of the central channel mingles with the energies of the right and left channels and the commingled energies exit from the physical body to the etheric body at these points:

1.   From the end of the fingertips and the tips of the toes, extending to the boundary of the etheric body.
2.   From the bai hui point at the crown of the head to the boundary of the etheric body above the head, where one's own personal energy connects with the energy of heaven (cosmic energy).
3.   From the center of the ball of each foot extending out to below the feet, to the boundary of the etheric body beneath, where one's personal energy connects with the energy of the earth.

Figure 1: The Central Channel

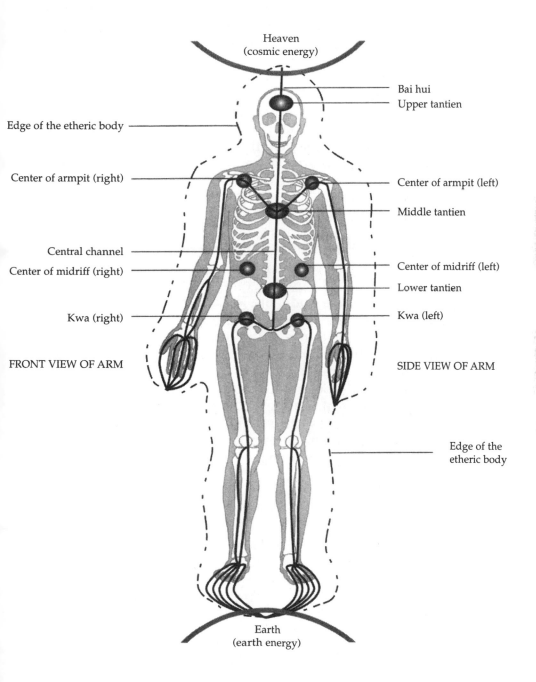

Heaven
(cosmic energy)

Bai hui
Upper tantien

Edge of the etheric body

Center of armpit (right)

Center of armpit (left)

Middle tantien

Central channel
Center of midriff (right)

Center of midriff (left)
Lower tantien

Kwa (right)

Kwa (left)

FRONT VIEW OF ARM

SIDE VIEW OF ARM

Edge of the
etheric body

Earth
(earth energy)

The Pathway of the Left and Right Channels

In the head and shoulders: From the crown of the head down to the collarbone, at no time do the left and right channels intersect the central channel. The left and right channels begin at the bai hui point at the crown of the head (where their energies are merged with that of the central channel). They continue down the center of the brain going parallel on either side of the central channel at an imperceptible distance away from it. At the upper tantien (third eye), the distance between the left and right channels widens, and they continue down to the center of the eyes, to the nostrils, down each side of the mouth, down the throat, to the level of the clavicals, close to but without intersecting the central channel. At this point the left and right channels branch off on a line to the left and to the right along the center line between the clavicals and back, where they join temporarily with the central channel in the center of the armpits, before splitting off again.

In the arms: From the center of the armpits on their respective sides of the body, the left and right channels run down each arm to the fingertips within the bone matrix (calicum) of both the bones of the arm and the joints to the ends of the five fingertips. Here, the left and right channels merge with the central channel.

In the legs: Beginning from the kwa (inguinal fold), both the left and right channels run within the bone matrix of their respective hip sockets, thigh and shin bones, knee and ankle joints, within the small bones of the feet along two thin parallel lines on either side of the central channel, to the center of the ball of the foot where the left right and central channels merge. They then split again and go to the tips of the toes, where again the left and right channels merge with the central channel and the commingled energy continues to the boundary of the etheric body.

The control gates of the left and right channels: There are three energetic "sluice gates" that either allow energy to pass unimpeded through the left and right channels or diminish it or completely cut off its flow. These are located in the center of the armpits, the center of the midriff, and the kwa.

Figure 2: The Left and Right Channels

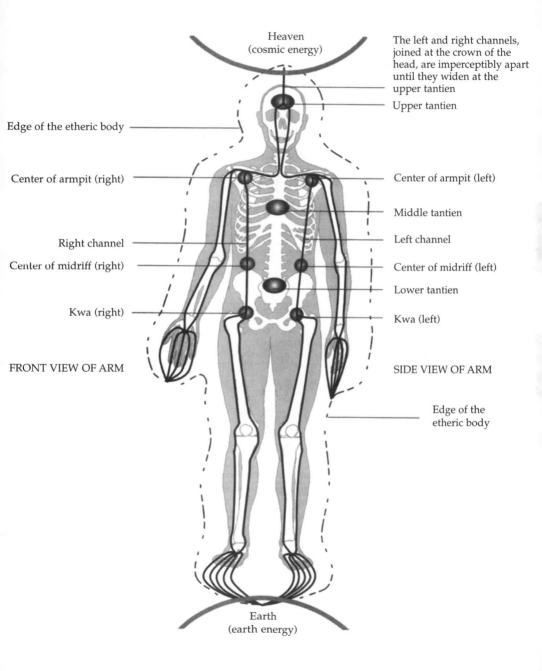

Heaven
(cosmic energy)

The left and right channels, joined at the crown of the head, are imperceptibly apart until they widen at the upper tantien

Upper tantien

Edge of the etheric body

Center of armpit (right)

Center of armpit (left)

Middle tantien

Left channel

Right channel

Center of midriff (right)

Center of midriff (left)

Lower tantien

Kwa (right)

Kwa (left)

FRONT VIEW OF ARM

SIDE VIEW OF ARM

Edge of the
etheric body

Earth
(earth energy)

The B. K. Frantzis Energy Arts® Program

(**Trainings Available**)

B. K. Frantzis and/or his trained instructors teach various aspects of Taoist Energy Arts in seminars, retreats, and classes at locations in North America and Europe. For information concerning instruction schedules, books, videos, and audiotapes, contact:

B. K. Frantzis Energy Arts®
P. O. Box 99
Fairfax, CA 94978-0099
USA
Phone: (415) 454-5243
Fax: (415) 454-0907
Web site: www.energyarts.com

The Six-Part Chi Gung Program

This program teaches the internal energy work of the 16 Taoist nei gung components (see Volume 1, *Relaxing Into Your Being*, p. 55). Together, these courses provide a complete chi gung regimen, combining the energy work of Oriental medicine, Taoist meditation, and physical movement.

The courses are:

Dragon and Tiger Chi Gung

This 1500-year-old traditional chi gung practice is a seven-movement exercise, ideal for any age or fitness level. Easy to learn, it quickly allows you to recognize the chi in your body and project/absorb energy from your hands. These techniques have been applied since antiquity to heal by clearing the blockages in human energy auras.

Opening the Energy Gates of Your Body

Learn to focus your awareness to consciously coordinate and control your body's flow of chi. *Energy Gates* teaches basic Taoist breathing, how to do standing chi gung, dissolve energy blockages, and feel your energy gates and their functions. You are taught to energize your internal organs and adjust internal biomechanical alignments to promote healing and begin to control the movements of your individual spinal vertebrae.

The Marriage of Heaven and Earth

This simple, one-movement exercise is widely used in China to relieve back, neck, joint, and neuromuscular problems. It is effective for increasing elasticity of the joints, overall strength, and upper-body flexibility. The openings and closings of the muscles (to induce the movement of energy through your acupuncture meridians) and the joints taught here are important internal techniques of Taoist martial arts for controlling chi.

Spinal Chi Gung: Bend the Bow and Shoot the Arrow

Learn the deepest level of Taoist breathing in which the spinal vertebrae, joints, cavities, glands and muscles physically and energetically link by expanding or contracting together with each breath. Learn how to fully control the multidirectional movement of all your vertebrae, correct back problems, and amplify your strength.

Spiraling Energy Body

Here, you learn to direct the upward flow of energy in your body, project your chi along spiraling pathways, open the right, left, and central energy channels, neutralize and transform negative energy, and direct energy at will to any point in your body.

Gods Playing in the Clouds

The six movements of *Gods* encompass all the internal techniques of chi gung. This powerful Taoist rejuvenation method amplifies all the material in the earlier chi gung courses. You also learn to make your bones harder, cleanse your emotional body of negative energy, and open and stabilize your heart center and central energy channel.

Meditation and Other Programs

Instruction is available in Taoist meditation, chi gung and tui na, as well as the internal martial arts of tai chi, hsing-i and ba gua. Instructor training programs are offered at various times. Write, call, fax, or visit our website for more information.

Please note: Mr Frantzis does not generally undertake one-on-one healings for specific problems. His time is currently devoted to instructing groups, training teachers, writing, and public health education.

Other Books By B. K. Frantzis

Opening the Energy Gates of Your Body
(North Atlantic Books)

The Power of Internal Martial Arts
(North Atlantic Books)

Relaxing Into Your Being–Reader's Edition
The Water Method of Taoist Meditation Series, Volume 1
(Available directly from B. K. Frantzis Energy Arts® only)

Videos

Taoist Energy Arts
In documentary style, this video shows and explains the key principles of chi gung, tai chi, chi bodywork, meditation and other Taoist preparatory practices. Included is rare footage of B. K. Frantzis' main teacher, the Taoist sage, Liu Hung Chieh, practicing in Beijing, China.
57 minutes.

Audiotapes

Chi Gung Dissolving
B. K. Frantzis explains the correct body alignments and breathing, for both standing and sitting dissolving. He provides guidelines for practice and leads you through the process of dissolving energy blocks.
66 minutes.

Other instructional videos and audiotapes available directly from:

B. K. Frantzis Energy Arts®
P. O. Box 99
Fairfax, CA 94978-0099
USA
Phone: (415) 454-5243
Fax: (415) 454-0907
Web site: www.energyarts.com